THE COMPLETE NECK PAIN SOLUTION

SUBTITLE:AN EVIDENCE-BASED GUIDE TO RELIEF AND LONG-TERM RECOVERY THROUGH TARGETED EXERCISES AND LIFESTYLE CHANGES

DR. K.D. CHRISTENSEN

CONTENTS

INTRODUCTION

As a retired Sports Chiropractor with over four decades of experience, I've witnessed countless patients struggle with the debilitating effects of neck pain. One particular case that stands out in my memory is that of Sarah, a young professional in her early thirties. When she first came to my clinic, Sarah was at her wit's end. The constant, nagging pain in her neck had begun to take over her life, affecting her work performance and straining her personal relationships.

Sarah's story is not unique. In fact, neck pain has become a pervasive issue in modern society. Studies show that up to 70% of adults will experience neck pain at some point in their lives, with many suffering from chronic or recurrent episodes. This widespread problem diminishes individuals' quality of life and takes a significant toll on productivity and healthcare systems worldwide.

Throughout my years of practice, I've come to understand that effective neck pain management requires a multifaceted approach. This book, "The Complete Neck Pain Solution," represents the culmination of my expertise and passion for helping people like

Sarah reclaim their lives from the grip of neck pain. By combining targeted exercises, lifestyle modifications, and mental wellness techniques, I've developed an evidence-based framework that empowers individuals to take control of their neck health.

My motivation for writing this book stems from a deep-rooted desire to share the knowledge and strategies I've honed over the years. Having worked with patients from all walks of life, from novice exercisers to seasoned athletes, I understand the unique challenges and frustrations that come with neck pain. This book is my way of reaching out to a wider audience, offering a comprehensive resource that can guide you towards sustainable relief and improved overall well-being.

As you embark on this journey, you'll gain a more in-depth understanding of your neck anatomy and the factors that contribute to pain. You'll learn how to implement targeted exercises, tailored to your fitness level, to strengthen and stabilize the muscles that support your neck. Additionally, you'll discover the crucial role that lifestyle modifications, such as posture correction and ergonomic adjustments, play in preventing and alleviating neck pain.

Throughout the book, you'll find clear, step-by-step instructions and visuals to ensure proper form and maximum benefit from each exercise. You'll also encounter real-life testimonials from individuals who have successfully navigated their own neck pain journeys, offering inspiration and proof that lasting relief is within reach.

Whether you're an adult seeking to reclaim your active lifestyle, an athlete looking to optimize your performance, or a young person aiming to establish healthy habits early on, this book is designed with you in mind. By engaging with the content and committing to the strategies outlined, you'll be well on your way to achieving a pain-free, more vibrant life.

As you progress through the chapters, I encourage you to take an active role in your recovery. Track your progress, celebrate your milestones, and remember that every small step forward is a victory worth acknowledging. With dedication and persistence, you'll alleviate your neck pain and cultivate a deeper sense of body awareness and self-care.

In the following pages, you'll find a roadmap to lasting neck pain relief. It's a journey that requires patience, commitment, and a willingness to embrace change. But rest assured, you don't have to navigate this path alone. As your guide and fellow traveler, I'll be with you every step of the way, sharing my expertise and support as you work towards a pain-free future.

So, let's begin this transformative journey together. With "The Complete Neck Pain Solution" as your companion, you're well-equipped to reclaim your life from the limitations of neck pain and discover a renewed sense of vitality and well-being.

1

UNDERSTANDING NECK PAIN AND ITS CAUSES

In the bustling world of modern life, neck pain often lurks like an unwelcome shadow, affecting countless individuals every day. You might recall a time when you woke up with a stiff neck, perhaps after a long day at your desk or an intense workout session. Such discomfort can be not only a nuisance but also a significant barrier to your daily activities and overall well-being. This chapter serves as a foundation for understanding the intricacies of neck pain, an essential step before diving into effective solutions. By exploring the anatomy of the neck, we aim to demystify the complex network of structures that enable movement and stability, providing you with a clearer picture of why neck pain occurs and how it can be managed. Through this understanding, you'll be better equipped to identify the root causes of your discomfort and take informed steps towards relief.

1.1 THE ANATOMY OF THE NECK: A SIMPLIFIED GUIDE

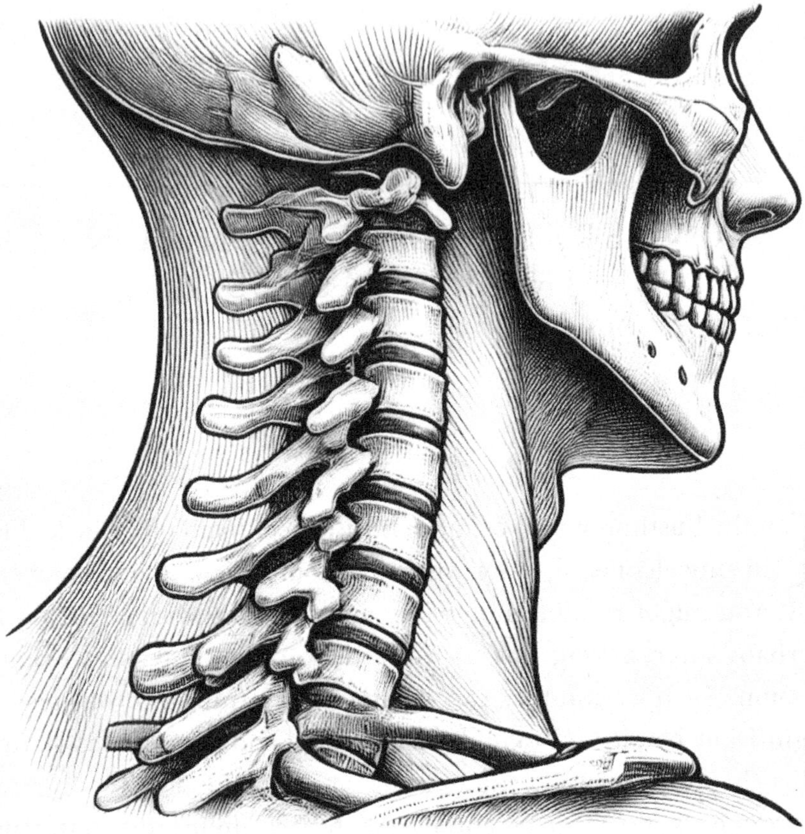

Fig 1.1 Cervical Spine Bony Anatomy

At the core of neck function lies the cervical spine, an elegant structure that supports your head and facilitates a remarkable range of motion. Comprised of seven vertebrae, labeled C1 through C7, the cervical spine connects your skull to your upper back. Each vertebra plays a crucial role, forming a protective tunnel for the spinal cord while allowing flexibility and strength. This intricate design enables movements such as flexion, where you tilt your chin downward, extension, as you gaze upward, and lateral flexion, bending your neck to the side. The cervical spine also facilitates rotation, allowing you to turn your head side to side. Together, these movements provide the flexibility necessary for daily activities.

Supporting the vertebrae are numerous muscles that stabilize and move the neck. Key players include the sternocleidomastoid, which allows you to rotate your head, and the trapezius, which helps with tilting and extending. These muscles work in concert with smaller, deeper muscles that maintain posture and balance. Meanwhile, a complex network of nerves originating from the spinal cord transmits signals that control movement and sensation. These nerve pathways are vital for relaying information and can become sources of pain if compressed or irritated.

Neck pain often arises when these anatomical structures are subjected to strain or injury. Intervertebral discs, which act as cushions between vertebrae, can become herniated or degenerate with age, leading to discomfort and reduced flexibility. Ligaments, the tough bands of tissue that stabilize the cervical spine, can sprain when overstressed, causing pain and inflammation. Such injuries disrupt the harmony of neck function, leading to the stiffness and soreness many experience daily.

Visual aids can greatly enhance your understanding of these structures, offering a clearer view of how the neck is composed and functions. Diagrams or illustrations can help you visualize the cervical spine, muscles, and nerves in relation to each other, providing a comprehensive understanding of the neck's architecture. This clarity is crucial in grasping how various elements can become sources of pain and dysfunction.

To make complex medical terms more accessible, it's important to translate them into everyday language. For instance, when discussing intervertebral disc issues, think of these discs as shock absorbers for your spine, allowing smooth, pain-free movement.

By simplifying terminology, we can bridge the gap between medical jargon and practical understanding, empowering you to take charge of your neck health. As you progress through this chapter, keep this anatomical framework in mind, as it will serve as the basis for identifying potential causes of neck pain and exploring targeted solutions.

1.2 COMMON CAUSES OF NECK PAIN: FROM TECH NECK TO STRESS

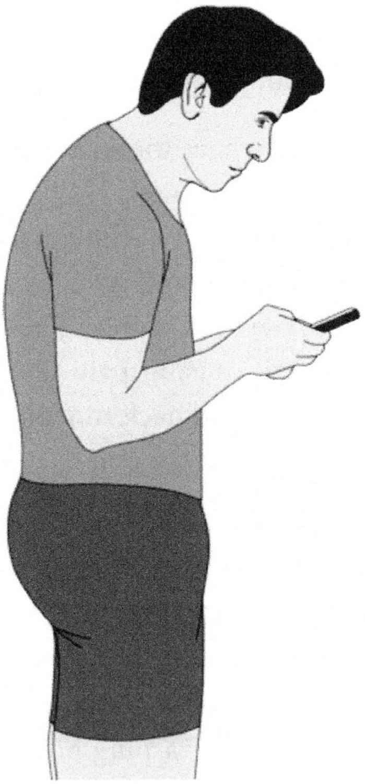

Fig 1.2 Tech Neck

In today's rapidly evolving digital age, our daily routines have shifted substantially, bringing with them modern lifestyle contributors to neck pain that were virtually unheard of just a few decades ago. One such pervasive issue is "tech neck," a condition stemming from the frequent use of smartphones, tablets, and computers. As we engage with our devices, whether it be scrolling through social media, responding to emails, or reading the latest news, we often find ourselves positioning our necks forward. This posture, where the head tilts forward at a sharp angle, places an undue amount of stress on the cervical spine, intensifying the pressure on our neck muscles and ligaments. The average adult head weighs approximately 10 to 12 pounds, and when angled forward, this weight increases, creating a significant burden that our necks must bear. Over time, this repetitive strain can lead to chronic pain, soreness, and even more severe musculoskeletal issues. Considering that people spend over three hours a day on their phones, the cumulative effect is substantial, making tech neck a modern epidemic.

Beyond the technological influences, our sedentary lifestyles further exacerbate neck pain issues. Many of us spend prolonged periods sitting at desks, commuting in cars, or lounging on couches, often in positions that do not support proper spinal alignment. This lack of movement can lead to muscle stiffness and weaken the supportive structures of the neck, setting the stage for discomfort and pain. Additionally, activities we might not immediately associate with neck pain, such as reading in bed with poor lighting or cradling a phone between the shoulder and ear, can also contribute to strain. These seemingly innocuous habits accumulate over time, manifesting as chronic pain that affects our daily functioning.

In addition to these lifestyle factors, certain physical contributors play a significant role in neck pain. Poor posture during daily activities, whether due to improper seating arrangements or simply inattentiveness, can lead to misalignment and muscle fatigue. Previous injuries, such as whiplash or sports-related traumas, may also predispose individuals to chronic neck issues. These injuries can create lasting damage to the cervical spine or surrounding tissues, leading to ongoing pain and discomfort. Repetitive strain injuries (RSI), often associated with tasks that require repetitive motions or sustained awkward positions, further compound these problems, as they lead to inflammation and irritation of muscles and tendons.

Psychological factors must not be overlooked, as they hold substantial sway over the physical manifestations of neck pain. Stress, a ubiquitous element of modern life, often triggers muscle tension through the release of stress hormones like cortisol. This tension can localize in the neck and shoulders, leading to stiffness and soreness. The mind-body connection is profound, with emotional stress frequently manifesting as physical discomfort. When individuals face high-pressure situations or experience anxiety, their muscles instinctively tighten, a natural response that becomes problematic when it persists over time. This tension not only exacerbates existing pain but can also lower pain tolerance, making even minor discomfort feel overwhelming.

The intricate nature of neck pain means it seldom arises from a single source. It is often a tapestry woven from various contributing factors, both physical and psychological. Understanding this multifactorial nature is crucial for effective management and relief. Recognizing the interplay between technology use, lifestyle habits, past injuries, and psychological stressors can provide a clearer picture of why neck pain occurs and how best to address it. By acknowledging the complexity of these issues, we can better tailor our approaches to prevention and treatment, paving the way for more effective strategies to alleviate neck discomfort.

1.3 IDENTIFYING YOUR PAIN: HOW TO RECOGNIZE SYMPTOMS AND TRIGGERS

Recognizing the nuances of neck pain can often feel like solving a complex puzzle, where each piece represents a different symptom or trigger. To effectively address your discomfort, it's crucial to first identify these elements through careful observation and reflection. One valuable tool in this process is a pain diary. By documenting your daily activities alongside your pain levels, you can uncover patterns that may not be immediately obvious. Consider noting the time of day when your neck pain intensifies, as well as any specific activities or positions that seem to exacerbate it. For instance, you might find that prolonged periods at your computer coincide with increased stiffness, or that a particular sleeping position leads to morning discomfort. These insights can reveal hidden triggers, serving as a roadmap for modifications in your routine.

Tracking your activities and their effects on your neck can be enlightening. Through this method, you start to see correlations between what you do and how you feel. This could involve noting how your neck responds to different exercises, or how stress levels impact your pain. For example, you might discover that a high-stress day at work correlates with increased tension and headaches. By pinpointing these connections, you not only gain a clearer understanding of your triggers but also open a pathway to more targeted and effective interventions.

Differentiating between types of neck pain is another critical step in understanding your condition. Pain can manifest in various forms, each offering clues about its underlying cause. Sharp pain, for instance, often signals an acute issue, such as a muscle strain or a pinched nerve. This type of pain tends to be sudden and intense, commonly resulting from a specific injury or movement. In contrast, dull pain might indicate chronic conditions, where the discomfort is more constant and less severe, often stemming from long-term issues like arthritis or muscle tension. Recognizing the character of your pain can guide your approach to treatment, helping you choose the most appropriate strategies for relief.

Radiating pain, where discomfort spreads from the neck to the shoulders, arms, or even hands, may suggest nerve involvement. This phenomenon, known as referred pain, occurs when nerves in the neck are compressed or irritated, sending pain signals to other parts of the body. Understanding these distinctions can be crucial in determining the appropriate course of action, as different types of pain often require varied interventions.

Common symptoms, like morning stiffness or headaches, can also provide valuable insights. Morning stiffness can suggest issues with sleeping posture or bed setup, indicating a need to evaluate your mattress or pillow. Headaches, particularly those starting at the base of the skull, may be linked to tension in the neck muscles. Such headaches often arise from poor posture or stress, highlighting the importance of addressing these factors in your daily life.

While self-assessment is a powerful tool, it's important to recognize when professional consultation is necessary. Persistent or severe symptoms, such as continuous sharp pain, numbness, or weakness, warrant a visit to a healthcare professional. Consulting with a chiropractor, physiotherapist, or physician can provide a more comprehensive evaluation, including diagnostic tools like X-rays or MRIs to uncover underlying issues. These experts can offer tailored advice and treatment plans, ensuring that you receive the most effective care for your specific condition.

Through this blend of self-assessment and professional guidance, you can develop a nuanced understanding of your neck pain, paving the way for informed decisions and targeted relief. By taking an active role in recognizing your symptoms and triggers, you empower yourself to make meaningful changes that can significantly improve your quality of life.

1.4 THE ROLE OF POSTURE: HOW EVERYDAY HABITS AFFECT YOUR NECK

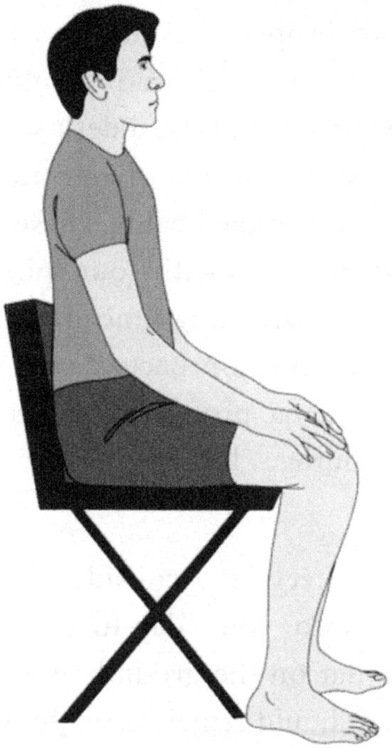

Fig 1.3 Correct sitting posture

Posture serves as the silent architect of your neck's health, sculpting either a structure of resilience or one of vulnerability. Our daily habits, often unconscious, can leave a lasting imprint on the alignment and function of our cervical spine. Slouching, for instance, is a common posture pitfall. When you slouch, your head juts forward, shifting the load from your spine to your neck muscles. This forward head posture places immense strain on the cervical spine, disrupting its natural curvature and leading to muscle fatigue and tension. Over time, this habitual misalignment can exacerbate neck pain and contribute to degenerative changes in the spine. It's a posture that many adopt without realizing its insidious effects, especially during long hours at a desk or while engrossed in a smartphone or laptop.

Ergonomics plays an indispensable role in mitigating the adverse effects of poor posture. Proper workstation setup can significantly alleviate the strain on your neck and shoulders. An ergonomic chair that supports your lower back, a desk set at the right height, and a monitor positioned at eye level can transform your workspace into a sanctuary for spinal health. These adjustments ensure that your neck remains aligned with your spine, reducing the risk of musculoskeletal stress. Investing time and effort into setting up an ergonomic workstation is a proactive step towards preserving neck health and enhancing productivity. It's about creating an environment that encourages healthy posture as a natural part of your daily routine.

To improve posture effectively, consider incorporating simple corrective strategies into your day-to-day life. When sitting, ensure your feet are flat on the ground, and your knees are at a right angle. Your back should remain straight, with your shoulders relaxed and pulled back. Standing posture is equally important: distribute your weight evenly on both feet, and align your ears with your shoulders while keeping your chin parallel to the floor. Adding exercises that counteract poor posture can also be beneficial. Shoulder blade squeezes, neck stretches, and core strengthening exercises can all contribute to better alignment. These activities, though seemingly minor, can make a significant difference in how your neck feels and functions.

The pervasive influence of technology on posture cannot be overlooked. Many spend hours each day interacting with devices, often in positions that compromise spinal integrity. To combat this, adjust your screen height so it remains at eye level, preventing the neck from craning forward. Maintain a viewing distance of about 20-30 inches, allowing a comfortable and natural gaze. When using handheld devices, bring them to eye level rather than bending your head down. These small modifications go a long way in maintaining a neutral posture, reducing the risk of tech-related neck strain.

Embracing good posture offers long-term benefits that extend beyond immediate comfort. By maintaining proper alignment, you safeguard your neck against the wear and tear that leads to chronic pain and dysfunction. Good posture supports the natural curvature of your spine, distributing weight evenly and reducing stress on muscles and ligaments. This prevents pain and enhances your overall physical function. Over time, consistent attention to posture can improve your body's biomechanics, leading to more efficient movement patterns and a reduced risk of injury. The commitment to good posture is a commitment to long-term wellness, offering a foundation for a healthy, pain-free life.

1.5 STRESS AND NECK PAIN: UNDERSTANDING THE CONNECTION

Stress is an omnipresent force, weaving its way into the fabric of our daily lives, and its impact on our physical health, particularly neck pain, is profound. Many people might be surprised to learn just how deeply intertwined stress and neck pain can be. This connection is largely due to the effects of stress hormones like cortisol, which, when released in excess, prompt muscles to contract and tighten. This involuntary response, often referred to as muscle tension, is particularly pronounced in the neck and shoulders, areas that commonly bear the brunt of our emotional burdens. Consider a typical day where deadlines loom, and personal responsibilities stack up. The weight of these pressures doesn't just rest on your mind; it manifests physically, often as a stiff neck or aching shoulders, creeping in without warning.

Emotional stress, though intangible, finds a physical foothold within us. When we're anxious or overwhelmed, our bodies react, tightening muscles as if bracing against an unseen threat. This tension can exacerbate existing neck pain or spark new episodes of discomfort, creating a vicious cycle where pain leads to stress, which in turn intensifies the pain. The body's heightened state of alertness reduces its ability to relax, and the prolonged muscle tension can lead to inflammation and soreness. This cycle can severely impact one's quality of life, limiting the range of motion and making even simple tasks burdensome.

To combat the impact of stress on neck pain, incorporating stress management techniques into your daily routine can make a significant difference. Breathing exercises are a simple yet powerful tool to foster relaxation and alleviate tension. By focusing on deep, rhythmic breathing, you can activate the body's parasympathetic nervous system, which helps calm the mind and relax muscles. Mindfulness and meditation practices offer another avenue for stress reduction. These techniques encourage a state of awareness and presence, helping to dissolve stress before it takes a physical toll. By dedicating a few minutes each day to mindfulness, you can cultivate a buffer against the stressors that contribute to neck pain.

Real-life examples of individuals who have successfully integrated stress management into their lives illustrate the potential benefits. Take, for instance, a corporate executive who attributed her chronic neck pain to the relentless demands of her job. By adopting a daily routine of meditation and controlled breathing, she found relief from her physical symptoms and gained a newfound resilience against workplace pressures. Her story exemplifies how addressing the root causes of stress can lead to tangible improvements in physical health.

Holistic approaches, which combine stress management with physical treatments, are particularly effective. Integrating relaxation techniques with physical therapies, such as chiropractic adjustments or physiotherapy, provides a dual approach to managing neck pain. This combination addresses both the physical and psychological components of pain, offering a more rounded and effective solution. By considering the mind and body as interconnected, you can develop a more comprehensive strategy for relief.

Incorporating these practices into your routine doesn't require a drastic lifestyle overhaul. Instead, small, consistent changes can yield significant benefits. A few minutes of deep breathing during a lunch break or a short meditation session before bed can help mitigate the effects of stress. Over time, these practices reduce neck pain and enhance overall well-being, fostering a sense of balance and calm amidst the chaos of everyday life.

1.6 WHEN TO SEEK PROFESSIONAL HELP: RECOGNIZING SERIOUS SYMPTOMS

Understanding when to seek professional help for neck pain is crucial, as it can prevent minor issues from escalating into chronic conditions. Persistent pain, despite your best self-care efforts, is a significant red flag. If you've tried various home remedies, from heat and cold therapy to exercise modifications, and the pain remains unabated, it might be time to consult a healthcare professional. Ignoring persistent pain can lead to complications, making early intervention vital for successful treatment outcomes.

Additionally, if you experience numbness, tingling, or weakness in your limbs, these symptoms could indicate nerve involvement, possibly due to a herniated disc pressing on a nerve. This situation can lead to more severe issues if left untreated. Sudden, severe neck pain, especially if it follows an injury or accident, should never be ignored. Such pain might suggest a serious underlying condition, such as a fracture or significant ligament damage, requiring immediate medical attention by an orthopedic spine specialist.

Once you've decided to seek professional help, knowing which specialist to consult can streamline the process. Chiropractors are often the first point of contact for structural adjustments. Chiropractic advice can be invaluable, particularly for issues related to spinal alignment and nerve pressure. Chiropractors offer non-surgical solutions that complement your recovery plan, providing relief and improving overall function. Chiropractors specializing in not only adjustments but exercise recovery include:

- American Chiropractic Board of Sports Physicians™: https://www.acbsp.com/directory/
- American Chiropractic Rehabilitation Board: https://acrb.org/location/

Physical therapists play a crucial role in rehabilitation, offering exercises and techniques to strengthen the neck, improve flexibility, and prevent future injuries. Their expertise in movement and exercise science allows them to design personalized rehab programs that address individual needs, promoting long-term recovery. Consulting these specialists can provide targeted interventions that address both the symptoms and root causes of neck pain.

As you prepare to visit a healthcare provider, familiarizing yourself with potential diagnostic procedures can reduce anxiety and help you engage more actively in your care. MRI and X-ray evaluations are common tools used to visualize the spine's structure and identify abnormalities, such as disc herniations, fractures, or degenerative changes. These imaging techniques provide detailed insights, guiding treatment decisions and ensuring that interventions are appropriately tailored to your condition.

Active participation in your healthcare journey is empowering. By understanding the potential causes of your pain and the diagnostic tools available, you can communicate more effectively with your healthcare provider. Ask questions, seek clarification, and discuss treatment options thoroughly. This collaborative approach ensures that your care plan aligns with your goals and preferences, enhancing the likelihood of a successful outcome.

Recognizing the signs that warrant professional evaluation is a vital component of neck pain management. By staying vigilant for persistent pain, neurological symptoms, and sudden severe discomfort, you can take timely action to address these issues. Consulting with the right specialists and understanding the diagnostic process empowers you to make informed decisions about your health. Engaging actively with your care facilitates recovery and fosters a proactive stance toward maintaining neck health. Taking these steps ensures that you're not just reacting to pain, but actively working toward a healthier, pain-free life.

2

LIFESTYLE ADJUSTMENTS FOR LONG-TERM RELIEF

Imagine stepping into an office where the hum of computers is constant, and the pace is relentless. Among the sea of desks, you notice one particular setup that stands out. It's not just the sleekness of the equipment that draws your attention, but the person working there—their posture is impeccable, their movements fluid and unstrained. This scene might seem aspirational, yet it encapsulates the profound impact of an ergonomic workspace. Creating an environment that prioritizes your body's natural alignment is not just an option; it's a necessity. As we delve into the intricacies of designing a neck-friendly workspace, you'll discover practical strategies that transform your daily routine into a foundation for health and productivity.

Ergonomic workspace design is more than just a buzzword—it's a critical component in the prevention of neck strain. The way you set up your workstation can either alleviate or exacerbate discomfort. Start with your monitor. Ideally, the top of your screen should be at or slightly below eye level, about an arm's length away. This positioning minimizes the need for tilting or straining, promoting a natural, relaxed posture. Your chair plays an equally vital role. An ergonomic chair supports the natural curve of your spine, particularly the cervical region, reducing muscle stress. Features like adjustable lumbar support and customizable height are essential. They allow you to tailor the chair to your unique needs, ensuring that your feet rest flat on the floor and your knees are at a right angle, fostering an environment of comfort and support.

Incorporating specific ergonomic tips can further enhance your workspace. Consider investing in an ergonomic keyboard and mouse. These tools are designed to keep your wrists and hands in a neutral position, reducing strain and preventing repetitive stress injuries. Position your phone and other frequently used items within easy reach. This minimizes twisting and reaching, movements that can lead to muscle tension. The goal is to create a seamless workflow where each component supports your body's natural mechanics, reducing the risk of strain and injury.

Standing desks have gained popularity for their ability to promote neck health. These adjustable desks allow you to alternate between sitting and standing, encouraging movement and preventing the stiffness that comes from prolonged sitting. When using a standing desk, maintain proper alignment: stand with your feet shoulder-width apart, distribute your weight evenly, and keep your head aligned with your spine. Transition between sitting and standing every 30 minutes to an hour. This variability not only benefits your neck but also enhances circulation and energy levels.

The concept of micro-breaks is a simple yet effective strategy to reduce neck strain. These short, frequent breaks remind you to step away from your desk and stretch your body. Incorporate stretching exercises that target the neck and shoulders. Simple movements, such as gentle neck rolls and shoulder shrugs, can alleviate tension and promote relaxation. These breaks, though brief, provide an opportunity to reset your posture and refresh your mind, ultimately boosting productivity and well-being.

Interactive Element: Ergonomic Workspace Checklist

- **Monitor Height**: Ensure the top of your screen is at or slightly below eye level.
- **Chair Adjustments**: Use an ergonomic chair with adjustable lumbar support.
- **Keyboard and Mouse**: Invest in ergonomic models to maintain wrist neutrality.
- **Item Positioning**: Keep frequently used items within easy reach.
- **Standing Desk**: Alternate between sitting and standing every 30-60 minutes.
- **Micro-Breaks**: Schedule short breaks to stretch and reset posture.

Implementing these ergonomic principles can make a world of difference in your daily comfort and long-term neck health. By prioritizing your body's needs through thoughtful workspace design, you're taking a proactive step towards a healthier, more productive lifestyle.

2.1 THE IMPORTANCE OF SLEEP: CHOOSING THE RIGHT PILLOW AND POSITION

Sleep is a cornerstone of recovery and overall health, particularly when it comes to your neck. During sleep, your body repairs muscles and tissues, and your neck, often strained during the day, gets much-needed rest. Proper sleep supports spinal alignment, allowing ligaments and muscles to relax and heal. Adequate sleep also reduces inflammation and tension, crucial factors in alleviating neck pain. Yet, for many, the morning comes with stiffness and discomfort, often due to poor sleep choices. A key component in this equation is the pillow. The right pillow maintains the natural curve of your neck, providing support without forcing your spine into unnatural angles.

Selecting a pillow that supports neck alignment involves considering its type, firmness, and height. Memory foam pillows conform to the shape of your head and neck, offering personalized support. Cervical contour pillows have a unique design that cradles the neck while supporting the head, ideal for maintaining alignment. Adjustable pillows allow you to customize loft and firmness, adapting to your specific needs. The height of your pillow should keep your neck aligned with your spine, whether you're lying on your back or side. A pillow that is too high or too low can strain muscles and misalign the vertebrae, contributing to pain and discomfort. More information can be found at: https://www.footlevelers.com/products/orthopedic-pillows.

Your sleep position plays a pivotal role in neck health as well. Side sleeping is often recommended, with a pillow placed between your knees to maintain spinal alignment and reduce strain on your lower back. This position, combined with a supportive neck pillow, helps keep your spine straight. For back sleepers, a pillow that supports the natural curve of your neck is essential, while stomach sleeping is generally discouraged due to the unnatural twist it causes in the neck. If you're accustomed to sleeping on your stomach, gradually transitioning to a side or back position can alleviate pressure on your cervical spine and promote better alignment.

Creating an environment conducive to restful sleep is equally important. Sleep hygiene refers to the practices and conditions that promote quality sleep, and it begins with your bedroom environment. Keep your room cool, as a lower temperature facilitates deeper sleep. Aim for a range between 60 and 67 degrees Fahrenheit, which is optimal for most people. Adjust lighting so that it's dim and soothing, as bright lights can disrupt your circadian rhythm. Blackout curtains or a sleep mask can block out light, enhancing your sleep quality. Additionally, consider the noise level in your room. White noise machines or earplugs can minimize disruptions, ensuring a peaceful environment.

The importance of sleep cannot be understated, especially when it comes to alleviating neck pain. By focusing on the right pillow, optimal sleep positions, and a conducive sleep environment, you take proactive steps towards better neck health. These choices, although seemingly simple, play a crucial role in how you feel each day, impacting not only your physical comfort but also your mental clarity and overall well-being.

2.2 REDUCING SCREEN TIME: PRACTICAL TIPS FOR LIMITING DEVICE USE

In today's digital landscape, screens have become ubiquitous, seamlessly integrating into almost every aspect of our lives. Whether it's checking emails, scrolling through social media, or binge-watching the latest series, our devices are constant companions. However, this increased screen time comes with a hidden cost, particularly for neck health. The posture often assumed during extended device usage—head tilted forward, shoulders slumped—places significant strain on the cervical spine. This position, colloquially known as "tech neck," results in increased pressure on the neck muscles, leading to discomfort and potential long-term damage. The repetitive nature of this strain can exacerbate existing neck issues, turning minor aches into chronic pain.

To counteract the negative effects of excessive screen time, implementing strategies to reduce device usage is crucial. One effective approach is to schedule regular digital detox periods. These breaks from screens not only give your eyes and neck a rest but also provide an opportunity to recharge mentally. Consider setting specific times each day when you step away from all devices. Whether it's during meals, an hour before bed, or a designated "tech-free" day each week, these breaks can significantly reduce the cumulative strain on your neck. Additionally, setting screen time limits on your devices can serve as a gentle reminder to take breaks. Most smartphones and tablets have built-in features that allow you to track usage and set daily limits. By consciously monitoring screen time, you can cultivate healthier habits that prioritize neck health.

Finding engaging alternatives to screen time can further support this endeavor. Outdoor hobbies such as walking or cycling not only offer physical benefits but also promote mental clarity and relaxation. These activities encourage you to engage with your environment, fostering a connection with nature that screens can't replicate. The rhythmic motion of walking or cycling can alleviate muscle tension, while the fresh air and natural surroundings enhance your overall well-being. Even simple activities like gardening or playing a sport can replace screen time, providing a dual benefit of physical exercise and mental rejuvenation.

Mindful technology use is another essential component of reducing screen time. This approach involves setting intentional purposes for device use, transforming mindless scrolling into deliberate action. Before reaching for your phone, ask yourself if the task at hand requires immediate attention or if it can wait. Designate specific times for checking emails or social media, allowing you to engage without the constant pull of notifications. By being purposeful in your interactions with technology, you can minimize unnecessary usage and focus on activities that truly matter. This conscious engagement fosters a healthier relationship with devices, reducing the habitual neck strain associated with excessive screen use.

Incorporating these strategies into your daily routine not only safeguards your neck health but also enriches your overall lifestyle. By reducing screen time and embracing alternative activities, you create a balanced approach to technology use that promotes physical and mental well-being. This shift allows you to reclaim time for activities that nurture your body and mind, ultimately leading to a more fulfilling, less strained existence.

2.3 MINDFULNESS AND STRESS REDUCTION TECHNIQUES FOR NECK PAIN

In the intricate dance of daily life, stress often takes the lead, pulling us into a rhythm that strains both mind and body. For those grappling with neck pain, this stress manifests all too often as tension and discomfort. Mindfulness emerges as a powerful tool in this scenario, offering relief by anchoring us in the present and easing the physical burdens we carry. Imagine starting your day with a simple practice: mindful breathing. By focusing on each inhale and exhale, you invite relaxation into tense muscles. This practice isn't just about breathing; it's about creating space to release what no longer serves you. As you breathe deeply, you activate the parasympathetic nervous system, a counterbalance to stress, which can help ease the tension in your neck and shoulders. Mindful breathing becomes a sanctuary, a moment where you step away from the chaos and nurture your well-being.

Another integral practice is the body scan meditation, where you systematically focus on different parts of your body, increasing awareness and connection. As you mentally scan from head to toe, you might notice areas of tension or discomfort that were previously unnoticed. This heightened awareness allows you to address tension before it escalates into pain. By regularly engaging in body scan meditation, you cultivate a more in-depth understanding of your body's signals, empowering you to make informed choices that support your neck health. This practice becomes a gentle reminder that your body and mind are partners in your well-being, working together to maintain balance and harmony.

Stress reduction techniques complement mindfulness practices by providing practical ways to manage tension. Progressive muscle relaxation is a straightforward method that involves tensing and then relaxing different muscle groups. This exercise reduces tension and improves your ability to recognize when muscles are tensed. By incorporating this technique into your routine, you create a proactive approach to managing stress and preventing neck pain. Imagine sitting comfortably, closing your eyes, and slowly tensing your shoulders, holding for a few seconds, then releasing. Feel the tension melt away, leaving relaxation in its wake. This deliberate cycle of tension and release teaches your muscles to respond to stress with ease rather than contraction.

Incorporating mindfulness into daily routines can transform everyday moments into opportunities for relaxation. Whether it's taking a mindful walk, savoring a cup of tea, or simply pausing for a few deep breaths, these practices weave tranquility into the fabric of your day. The mind-body connection is a powerful ally in this process. Mental well-being and physical health are intricately linked, each influencing the other. When you nurture your mental health, you simultaneously support your physical health, creating a positive feedback loop that fosters overall well-being. A calm mind promotes relaxed muscles, reducing the likelihood of tension-related neck pain.

Consistency is key when it comes to mindfulness and stress reduction. Regular practice enhances the effectiveness of these techniques and reinforces your commitment to self-care. Think of mindfulness as a muscle—the more you use it, the stronger it becomes. Over time, these practices become second nature, seamlessly integrated into your lifestyle. They become tools you can rely on when life's challenges threaten to disrupt your equilibrium. By making mindfulness a regular part of your routine, you build resilience against stress, empowering yourself to navigate life's ups and downs with grace and ease.

2.4 THE IMPACT OF NUTRITION: ANTI-INFLAMMATORY FOODS FOR NECK HEALTH

Diet plays a pivotal role in managing inflammation, a common culprit behind neck pain. What you eat can either fuel inflammation or combat it, influencing how your body feels each day. Foods high in sugar, refined carbs, and unhealthy fats are notorious for promoting inflammation. These include processed snacks, sugary beverages, and fried items, all of which can exacerbate pain and discomfort. On the other hand, incorporating anti-inflammatory foods into your diet provides a natural way to soothe and heal. These foods work by reducing the body's inflammatory responses, supporting overall health, and enhancing your well-being.

One of the most effective dietary additions for combating inflammation is fatty fish, rich in omega-3 fatty acids. Salmon, mackerel, and sardines are excellent choices, offering powerful anti-inflammatory properties that can help alleviate joint and muscle pain. Omega-3s are known for reducing the production of inflammatory cytokines, molecules that contribute to inflammation in the body. By incorporating these fish into your meals a few times a week, you can significantly improve your body's ability to manage inflammation.

Colorful fruits and vegetables are another dietary powerhouse for reducing inflammation. Berries, such as blueberries and strawberries, are loaded with antioxidants that protect your cells from damage and reduce inflammation. Leafy greens like spinach and kale are equally beneficial, offering a rich source of vitamins and minerals that support your immune system. The vibrant hues of these foods are not just pleasing to the eye; they indicate the presence of phytochemicals, compounds that fight inflammation and promote health. Regular consumption of a variety of these fruits and vegetables can enhance your body's resilience against pain and discomfort.

Nuts and seeds, including almonds, walnuts, and flaxseeds, are potent sources of healthy fats that combat inflammation. These foods provide essential nutrients, such as vitamin E and magnesium, which play a role in reducing inflammation and supporting neck health. Incorporating a handful of nuts into your daily diet can offer a satisfying crunch while also delivering anti-inflammatory benefits. Flaxseeds, in particular, are rich in alpha-linolenic acid, a type of omega-3 fatty acid that supports joint health. Adding these seeds to smoothies, yogurt, or salads is a simple way to enhance your meals with anti-inflammatory goodness.

Meal planning can make integrating these foods into your daily routine more manageable. Consider starting your day with a breakfast of oatmeal topped with berries and a sprinkle of flaxseeds. For lunch, a salad loaded with leafy greens, colorful vegetables, and grilled salmon can provide a satisfying and nutritious meal. Snack on a mix of nuts and seeds throughout the day to keep inflammation at bay. Dinners can feature dishes like roasted vegetables and fish, offering a balance of flavors and nutrients. By planning meals around these foods, you ensure a steady intake of anti-inflammatory nutrients that support neck health.

Hydration also plays a crucial role in maintaining overall health and managing inflammation. Water helps transport nutrients to your cells and supports the elimination of waste, keeping your body functioning optimally. Adequate hydration also aids in maintaining the health of your spine's intervertebral discs, which are essential for neck flexibility and comfort. Aim to drink enough water throughout the day, adjusting your intake based on activity level and climate. Herbal teas and water-rich foods, such as cucumbers and melons, can contribute to your hydration goals while offering additional health benefits.

2.5 SUSTAINABLE PRACTICES: ECO-FRIENDLY ADJUSTMENTS FOR A HEALTHIER NECK

Incorporating sustainability into your lifestyle is more than a trend; it's a commitment to your health and the planet's well-being. Sustainable practices contribute to environmental conservation and enhance personal health, including the health of your neck. By choosing eco-friendly ergonomic products, you can maintain alignment and reduce neck strain while minimizing your ecological footprint. These products are crafted with materials that are both durable and environmentally responsible. For instance, chairs made from recycled materials or desks designed with renewable resources offer the dual benefits of ergonomic support and sustainability. Such choices reflect a dedication to preserving the planet while taking care of your body.

Practical eco-friendly tips extend beyond the office. Consider the impact of everyday items like water bottles. Switching to reusable water bottles helps reduce waste and ensures you stay hydrated, which is essential for maintaining muscle health and elasticity.

This choice not only supports your neck health by keeping your body well-hydrated but also reduces the reliance on single-use plastics, significantly cutting down on environmental harm. Opting for sustainable materials in home and office furnishings is another step. Bamboo, for instance, is a renewable resource that is both sturdy and stylish, making it an excellent choice for furniture that supports good posture and neck health.

Outdoor activities play a significant role in promoting both physical and mental health. Engaging with nature offers a respite from the digital world, providing an opportunity to breathe fresh air and move your body in ways that support musculoskeletal health. Activities like hiking, gardening, or even simple nature walks not only help improve your neck strength and flexibility through natural movement but also reduce stress levels. These moments of connection with nature recalibrate your focus and foster a sense of peace and well-being, which in turn can alleviate neck tension. Additionally, these activities often require little to no equipment, which aligns with sustainable living by reducing resource consumption.

Sustainable living extends its benefits beyond the individual to the broader community and environment. By adopting eco-friendly practices, you contribute to a culture of sustainability that can inspire others within your community. This collective approach amplifies the positive impact, leading to healthier ecosystems and more resilient communities. Moreover, sustainable choices often support local and ethical businesses, further strengthening community ties and economic stability. The ripple effect of one person's sustainable choices can lead to significant environmental benefits, such as reduced pollution and conservation of natural resources. This interconnectedness between personal wellness and community health highlights the importance of sustainability as a shared responsibility.

As you integrate these sustainable practices into your life, you're not just making choices for today but investing in the future of your health and the planet. By prioritizing eco-friendly products, engaging in outdoor activities, and embracing sustainability in your daily routine, you create a holistic approach to neck health that extends beyond the physical. These practices promote a lifestyle that is conscious and considerate, fostering a connection between personal well-being and environmental stewardship. In this way, every decision you make becomes a step towards a healthier, more sustainable world. With a focus on sustainability, you set the foundation for a lifestyle that supports both your neck health and the planet's vitality. As you embrace these changes, consider how they align with the broader picture of maintaining balance in all aspects of life.

In the next chapter, we explore how targeted exercises can further enhance your neck health, building on the sustainable practices you've adopted. By combining these elements, you create a comprehensive strategy that supports long-term wellness.

3

TARGETED EXERCISES FOR NECK PAIN RELIEF

Imagine standing at the starting line of a race, your muscles tense and ready, the air electric with anticipation. Just as a runner must prepare their body for the challenge ahead, your neck requires a similar warm-up before delving into exercises designed to alleviate pain. Warming up is not merely a prelude to physical activity; it is a crucial step that primes your muscles, enhancing flexibility and blood flow. This preparation is vital for preventing injury and ensuring that each movement yields the maximum benefit, setting the stage for a successful exercise session.

Warming up increases blood flow to the neck muscles, a process that delivers oxygen and nutrients essential for optimal performance. This influx of blood prepares the muscles for action, reducing stiffness and enhancing joint mobility. Consider your neck as a finely tuned instrument: without a proper warm-up, the strings may be too tight, limiting their ability to produce the desired melody. Similarly, a neck unprepared for exercise is more susceptible to strain, which can exacerbate existing pain or create new issues. By dedicating time to this essential step, you lay the groundwork for a more effective and safer workout.

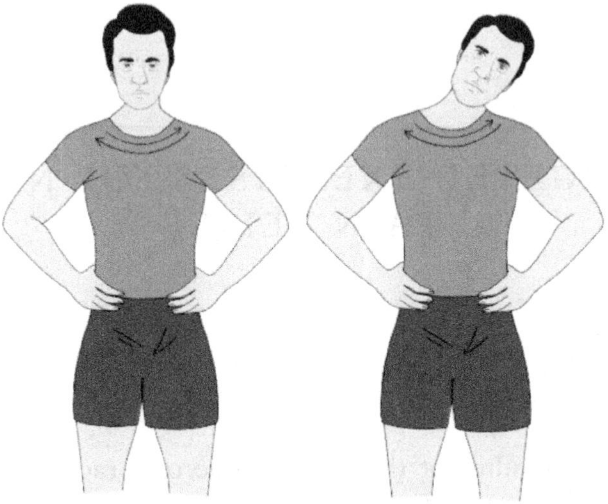

Fig 3.1 Neck Circles

Begin your warm-up with neck circles, a gentle exercise that loosens the muscles and promotes joint flexibility. Start with your head in a neutral position and slowly rotate it in a circular motion, as if drawing a circle in the air with your nose. Begin with small circles, gradually expanding the range as your muscles become more pliable. This exercise enhances flexibility and brings awareness to any areas of tension or discomfort, allowing you to adjust your movements accordingly. Neck circles are akin to a gentle massage, coaxing your muscles into a state of readiness without the risk of overextension.

Incorporate shoulder shrugs and rotations to further prepare your neck and upper body. With your arms relaxed at your sides, lift your shoulders towards your ears, hold for a moment, and release them back down. Follow this with shoulder rotations, moving your shoulders in a circular motion both forward and backward. These movements target the interconnected muscles of the neck and shoulders, promoting relaxation and enhancing blood flow. By engaging these areas, you set the stage for more intensive exercises, reducing the likelihood of strain or discomfort.

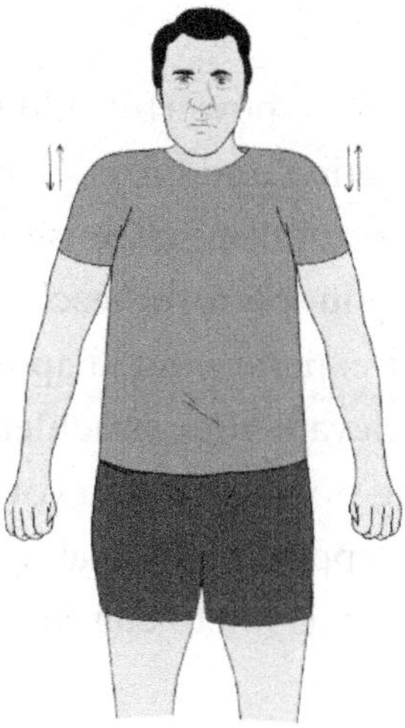

Fig 3.2 Shoulder Shrugs

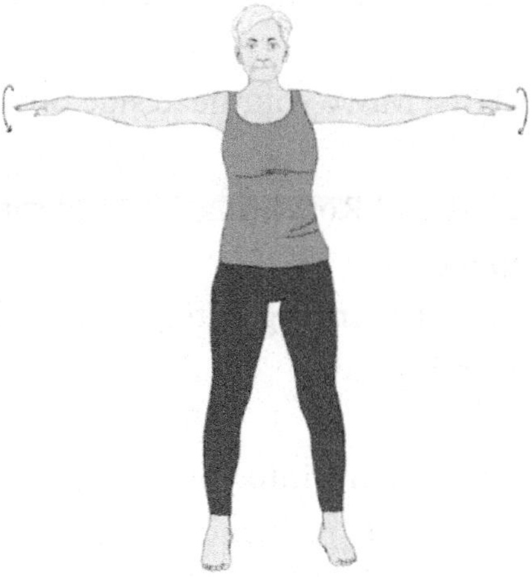

Fig 3.3 Shoulder Rotations

As you progress through your warm-up, pay attention to gradual progression. It's essential to start with gentle movements, allowing your body to acclimate before increasing intensity. Think of this process as waking up your muscles from a restful slumber, slowly coaxing them into action. By respecting this gradual approach, you ensure that your neck remains protected, minimizing the risk of injury.

Breathing techniques are a powerful addition to your warm-up routine, enhancing relaxation and focus. Deep breathing encourages the release of tension, promoting a sense of calm that permeates your entire body. As you perform each exercise, inhale deeply through your nose and expand your diaphragm while filling your lungs with air. Do not elevate your shoulders. Hold the breath for a moment before exhaling slowly through your mouth. This rhythmic diaphragm breathing supports physical relaxation and sharpens your mental focus, preparing you to engage fully with your exercises.

Interactive Element: Warm-Up Checklist

- **Neck Circles**: Start with small circles, gradually increasing in size.
- **Gentle Head Tilts**: Move your head side to side, feeling the stretch.
- **Shoulder Shrugs and Rotations**: Lift and rotate shoulders to warm up upper body.
- **Deep Diaphragm Breathing**: Integrate breathing with movements for relaxation.

By integrating these elements into your routine, you create a foundation of readiness and resilience. This preparation is not confined to physical benefits alone; it fosters a mindset of awareness and control, empowering you to approach your exercises with confidence. As you embark on this journey toward neck pain relief, remember that each warm-up is a step toward a stronger, more flexible, and pain-free you.

3.1 BEGINNER EXERCISES: GENTLE MOVEMENTS FOR NOVICES

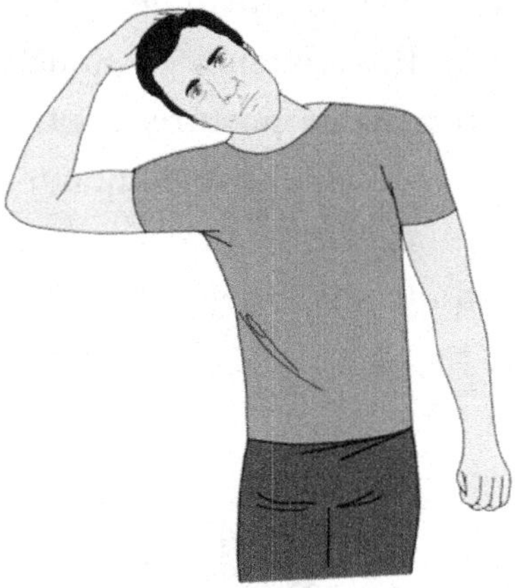

Fig 3.4 Neck Stretch

Starting a neck exercise routine can feel daunting, especially if you're new to addressing neck pain. However, beginning with simple, low-impact exercises can be incredibly beneficial. These gentle movements are designed to ease you into a routine without overwhelming your neck or causing additional strain. One such exercise is the neck stretch, which enhances flexibility. Slowly tilt your head towards one shoulder, reaching your opposite hand over your head to gently pull it further to the side. Hold this position for a few seconds, feeling the stretch along the side of your neck. Return to the center and repeat on the other side. This stretch increases flexibility and helps release tension built up from daily activities.

Chin tucks are another effective exercise, particularly for posture correction. With your back straight and shoulders relaxed, lay face up in a neutral position. Imagine a string pulling your head upward, elongating your spine. Gently draw your chin inward, as if attempting to create a double chin, while keeping your gaze forward. Hold this position briefly before releasing. This exercise strengthens the muscles that support your neck, promoting better alignment and reducing the tendency to slouch. Regular practice can significantly improve your posture, contributing to reduced neck pain over time. It's a small movement, but its impact on your neck's health is substantial, helping to counteract the forward head posture so common in our digital age. This same exercise can be performed sitting.

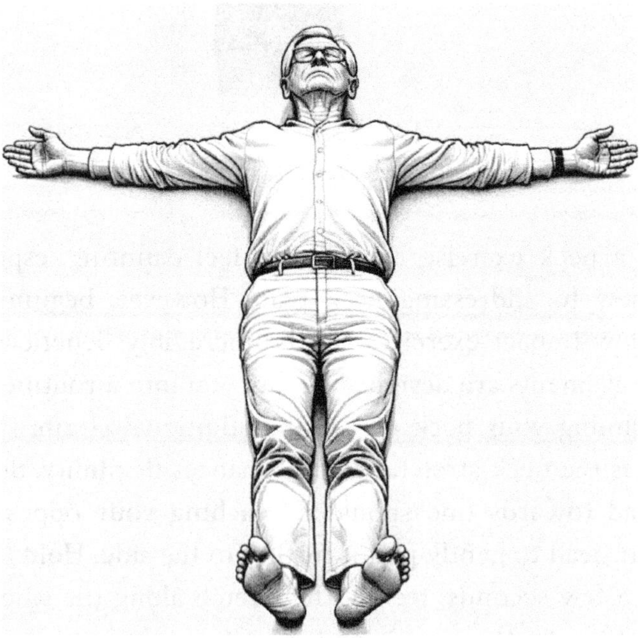

Fig 3.5 Chin Tucks

Proper form and alignment are crucial when performing neck exercises to prevent strain and maximize benefits. Always maintain a neutral spine, avoiding any excessive bending or twisting that could lead to injury. Imagine a straight line running from the top of your head down to your tailbone, and strive to keep this alignment throughout each exercise. Paying attention to form protects your neck and ensures that you engage the correct muscles, enhancing the effectiveness of each movement. It's about quality, not quantity; a few well-executed repetitions are far more beneficial than many performed with poor form.

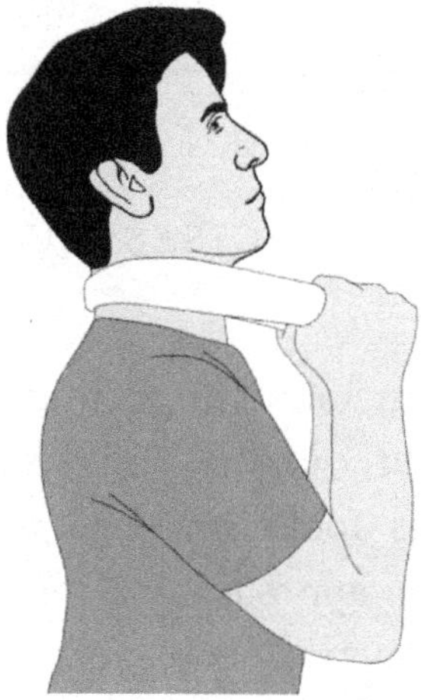

Fig 3.6 Towel Assisted Neck Extension

For those seeking additional support or modifications, using a towel during neck extensions can provide comfort and stability. Roll a towel lengthwise and place it behind your neck, holding the ends in each hand. As you gently extend your neck backward, use the towel for support, allowing it to guide your movement. This modification is particularly helpful if you're experiencing discomfort or if you're just beginning to explore neck exercises. It offers a controlled range of motion, ensuring that you don't overextend or strain your neck.

Consistency and patience are key when incorporating these exercises into your routine. It's important to remember that improvement takes time, and gradual progress is the most sustainable approach. Aim to practice these exercises regularly, ideally several times a week, to build strength and flexibility over time. While immediate results may be tempting, the true benefits of these exercises are realized through dedication and persistence. Embrace the process as an investment in your long-term neck health, and celebrate the small victories along the way, such as increased range of motion or reduced pain during daily activities. This steady commitment to your well-being will pay dividends, fostering a stronger, more resilient neck that supports you in all your endeavors.

3.2 INTERMEDIATE EXERCISES: BUILDING STRENGTH WITHOUT STRAIN

As you progress in your neck care routine, it's time to introduce moderate-intensity exercises that build strength while ensuring safety. These exercises focus on engaging neck muscles more deeply, yet they remain approachable for those ready to advance beyond the basics. Isometric neck exercises are a cornerstone of this approach. These involve contracting your neck muscles without actual movement, which effectively builds strength without risking strain. To perform an isometric neck exercise, sit or stand with your back straight. Place your right hand against the side of your head. Gently push your head into your hand while resisting the movement with your neck muscles. Hold for a few seconds before releasing. Repeat on the opposite side. This exercise engages the lateral neck muscles, fortifying them against future stress.

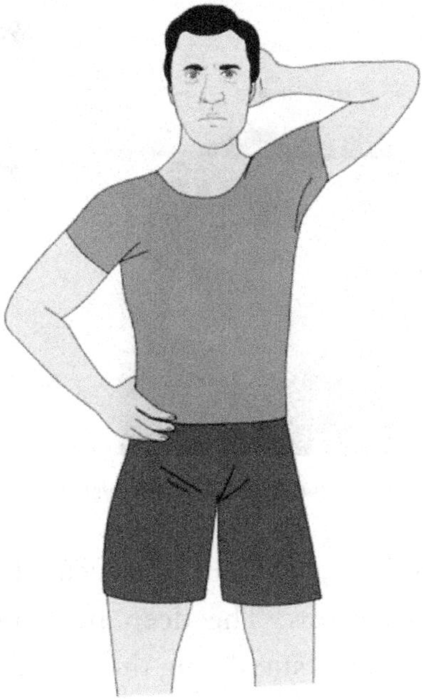

Fig 3.5 Isometric Neck Exercise

The **NECKSYS** Neck System is an important component of comprehensive cervical spine rehabilitation. It provides you with a simple way to perform prescribed exercises to enhance the effectiveness of cervical spine care. This exercise regime is meticulously designed to restore the integrity of the muscles supporting your neck, leading to significant improvements in your cervical posture. By focusing on isolated movements, it allows for a submaximal range of motion that is deliberately limited to avoid strain and promote healing. The program incorporates variable resistance, which can be adjusted to match your current strength level, ensuring a personalized approach to recovery. Additionally, the equipment required for these exercises can be easily mounted over a door, making it a convenient solution for both home and office settings. For more information: https://www.footlevelers.com/rehab/necksys

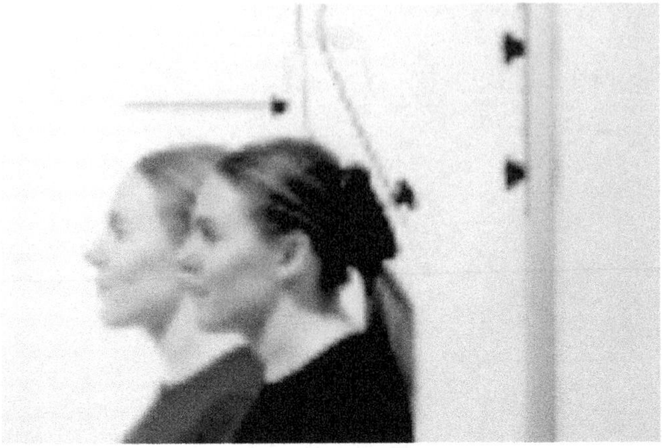

Fig 3.6 Necksys Neck System

Focusing on muscle engagement is crucial for maximizing the benefits of these exercises. The deep neck flexors, often overlooked, play a vital role in stabilizing the cervical spine. To activate these muscles, lie on your back with your knees bent and feet flat on the floor. Gently nod your chin as if signaling "yes," feeling the engagement at the front of your neck. This subtle movement strengthens the deep flexors, improving neck stability and posture. Consistent practice encourages these muscles to support the spine more effectively, reducing the likelihood of pain and discomfort.

Enhancing neck stability through balance and coordination drills is another key aspect of intermediate exercises. Stability ball exercises are particularly effective in this regard. Begin by sitting on a stability ball with your feet flat on the ground. Engage your core and slowly lift one foot off the ground, maintaining your balance. This simple act challenges your neck and core muscles to work in concert, fostering greater stability. As you gain confidence, you can incorporate additional movements, such as rotating your head from side to side while balancing. This enhances coordination, building a foundation of strength and resilience.

To ensure clarity and safety in these exercises, visual aids can be immensely helpful. Illustrations or video demonstrations can provide a clearer understanding of complex movements, guiding you through each step with precision. These resources can illustrate the correct form, highlight common mistakes, and offer tips for optimizing your practice. Accessing visual aids empowers you to perform each exercise correctly, maximizing benefits while minimizing the risk of injury.

3.3 ADVANCED NECK EXERCISES: FOR ATHLETES AND ACTIVE LIFESTYLES

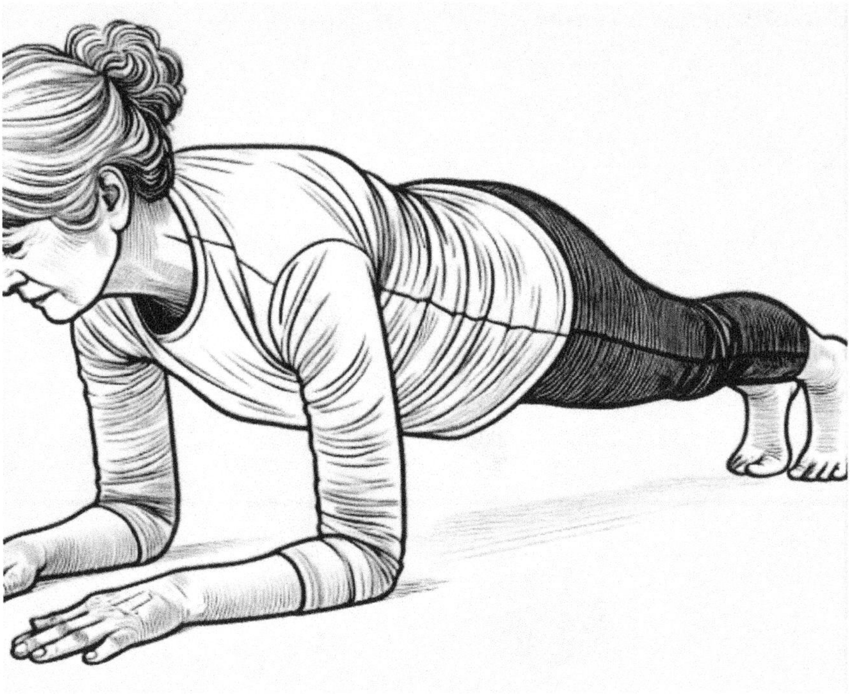

Fig 3.7 Plank with Chin Tuck

For those with an athletic background or a highly active lifestyle, the demands placed on the body, especially the neck, can be intense. Athletes often require a level of strength and flexibility that goes beyond the needs of the average individual. Engaging in advanced exercises helps in optimizing performance and in preventing potential injuries. One such exercise is the plank, a staple in core workouts, which can be modified to incorporate neck engagement. By simply adjusting your gaze and neck position during a plank, you can enhance the activation of stabilizing muscles. Assume a standard plank position, ensuring your body forms a straight line from head to heels. While maintaining this posture, gently draw your chin towards your chest, engaging the neck muscles without compromising the plank's integrity. This subtle modification fortifies the neck, integrating its strength into the core exercise routine.

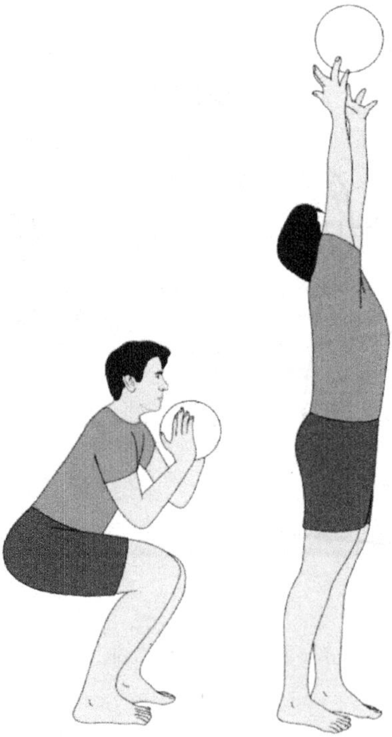

Fig 3.8 Plyometric exercise

Plyometric exercises introduce an element of dynamic strength, crucial for athletes who rely on explosive power. These exercises involve rapid and forceful movements that can be adapted to target neck strength. One method is to use a weighted ball or soft medicine ball. Hold the ball at chest level while standing upright. Slightly bend your knees, then explosively push the ball overhead while simultaneously extending the neck. This movement mimics the explosive actions often required in sports, enhancing both neck strength and coordination. As with all plyometrics, it's important to focus on controlled movements to prevent injury, ensuring that the explosive action is smooth and well-monitored.

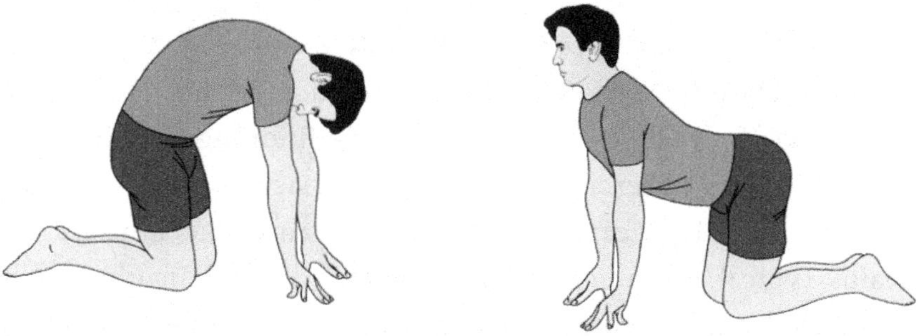

Fig 3.9 Camel Pose

Endurance and flexibility are equally critical for maintaining a well-rounded athletic profile. Advanced yoga poses, such as the Camel Pose or Fish Pose, specifically target the neck and shoulders, promoting increased flexibility and endurance. In the Camel Pose, kneel on the floor with your knees hip-width apart. Place your hands on your lower back for support, then slowly arch backward, reaching your hands towards your heels. This pose opens the chest and stretches the neck and shoulders, fostering greater range of motion and reducing the risk of stiffness.

Fish Pose, on the other hand, involves lying on your back and lifting your chest towards the ceiling while tilting your head backward. Both poses require mindful breathing to maximize the stretch, emphasizing a harmonious blend of strength and flexibility.

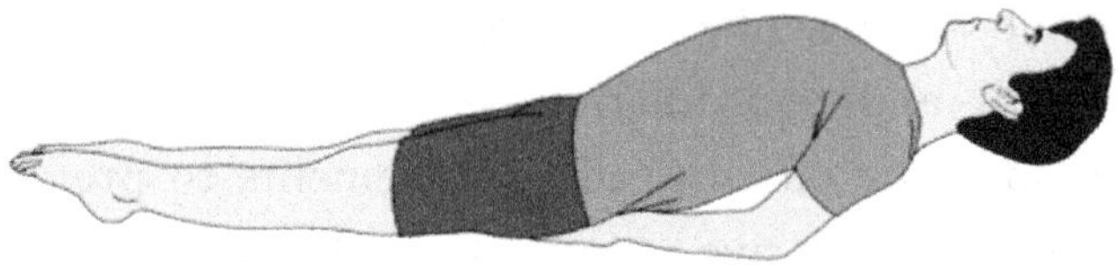

Fig 3.10 Fish Pose

Incorporating sport-specific drills into your regimen further tailors your exercise routine to your athletic pursuits. For contact sports like football or rugby, neck conditioning exercises are invaluable. These exercises simulate the physical demands encountered during play, fortifying the neck against the impacts and strains typical of these sports. An effective drill involves neck resistance training using a partner or resistance bands. Stand with your feet shoulder-width apart and place a band around your head. Have a partner hold the other end, providing resistance as you gently push forward, backward, and side-to-side with your neck. This resistance training promotes neck resilience, crucial for absorbing and managing the physical impacts experienced in competitive environments.

Safety remains paramount when engaging in advanced exercises. Monitoring for discomfort and adjusting intensity as needed is essential to prevent overexertion and injury. Pay close attention to how your neck responds during and after exercises. If you experience any sharp pain or unusual discomfort, it's important to reduce intensity or modify the exercise. Consistent evaluation and adjustment ensure that your workouts remain effective and safe, allowing you to push boundaries while respecting your body's signals.

3.4 FOAM ROLLING TECHNIQUES FOR NECK TENSION RELIEF

Imagine a tool that acts as both your massage therapist and physical therapist, all rolled into one. That's the beauty of foam rolling —a method that empowers you to tackle neck tension head-on with simplicity and precision. Foam rolling serves as a form of self-massage, targeting muscle tightness and promoting relaxation through myofascial release. Myofascial release involves applying pressure to the fascia, the connective tissue surrounding muscles, to alleviate pain and improve mobility. This technique can be particularly beneficial for the neck, where tension often accumulates due to stress and poor posture. By breaking up adhesions and increasing blood flow, foam rolling helps soothe sore areas and restore flexibility, making it a valuable addition to your neck care routine.

To begin your foam rolling practice, it's important to understand the proper technique to maximize benefits while minimizing the risk of injury. Start by selecting a foam roller that suits your comfort level—softer rollers provide gentler pressure, while firmer ones offer deeper release. Position the roller horizontally under your upper back, close to the base of your neck. Lie back slowly, supporting your head with your hands if needed, and use your feet to control the movement. Gently roll back and forth, allowing the roller to glide along your upper back and neck. This motion should be slow and controlled, focusing on areas that feel tense or tender. As you roll, remember to breathe deeply, which aids in relaxation and enhances the release of tension.

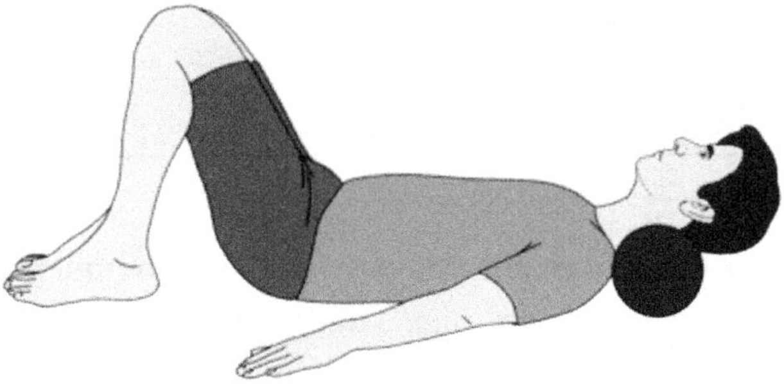

Fig 3.11 Neck Foam Rolling

Identifying the key areas to target is crucial for effective foam rolling. The trapezius muscles, which span across your shoulders and up to the base of your skull, are often a hotbed for tension. Similarly, the levator scapulae, which run along the sides of your neck, can become tight from prolonged sitting or stress. When you encounter a particularly tight spot, pause and apply gentle pressure for 20 to 30 seconds. This sustained pressure encourages the fascia to release, providing relief and improving range of motion. However, it's important to avoid applying pressure directly to the cervical spine, as this area requires gentle care to prevent injury. Focus instead on the muscles surrounding the neck, where tension is most likely to accumulate.

While foam rolling offers numerous benefits, it's essential to heed cautionary advice to ensure a safe and effective practice. Overuse can lead to muscle soreness or irritation, so limit your foam rolling sessions to a few times per week, especially when starting out. Foam rolling should be avoided during acute injury or if you experience sharp pain, as this may exacerbate the condition. Instead, allow time for healing and consult a healthcare professional for guidance. Always listen to your body and adjust the pressure and duration of your sessions as needed. If discomfort persists, seek advice from a qualified practitioner to ensure you're using the correct technique.

Understanding foam rolling's role in neck care can elevate your self-care routine, providing a practical and effective means of managing tension. Incorporating this technique into your regimen empowers you to take control of your neck health, offering relief from the strains of daily life. Whether you're an athlete looking to enhance performance or someone seeking relief from the rigors of desk work, foam rolling can be a valuable ally in your quest for a tension-free neck. By respecting its nuances and practicing with care, you can unlock the benefits of this versatile tool, paving the way for improved mobility and comfort.

3.5 ACTIVE RECOVERY: LOW-INTENSITY EXERCISES FOR ONGOING RELIEF

Active recovery is more than just a buzzword; it's a strategic approach to maintaining neck health through gentle, mindful movement. Unlike high-intensity workouts, active recovery focuses on promoting circulation and reducing muscle stiffness without overexertion. By keeping the body in motion, even at a low intensity, you encourage blood flow to the neck muscles, which aids in delivering essential nutrients and oxygen. This process helps to flush out metabolic waste, reducing stiffness and soreness that often follow more vigorous activities. Think of active recovery as a way to give your neck the care it needs while still keeping you engaged and active.

Incorporating low-intensity exercises into your routine can be both effective and enjoyable. Walking, for example, is a simple yet powerful activity that can be tailored to focus on posture and alignment. As you walk, pay attention to how you hold your head and shoulders, ensuring that your chin is parallel to the ground and your shoulders are relaxed. This supports your neck and enhances your overall posture. Another excellent choice is tai chi, an ancient practice known for its fluid, gentle movements. Tai chi encourages flexibility and balance, making it ideal for neck mobility. The slow, deliberate motions allow you to focus on the movement's quality rather than its intensity, fostering an environment of relaxation and healing.

To make active recovery part of your daily life, consider integrating these exercises into routine activities. Simple neck rolls can be seamlessly added to your morning routine, perhaps while you're brewing your coffee or waiting for your toast. These gentle movements help to loosen stiff muscles and set a positive tone for the day ahead. By making active recovery a consistent part of your daily habits, you reinforce the importance of regular movement, which can prevent stiffness from taking hold and maintain a sense of well-being.

While active recovery is beneficial, it's essential to balance it with adequate rest. Your body needs time to repair and recharge, especially after periods of exertion. Ensuring you get enough rest allows your muscles to recover fully, reducing the risk of overuse injuries. This balance between movement and rest creates a harmonious routine that supports long-term neck health. By listening to your body and respecting its need for both activity and downtime, you build a more sustainable approach to managing neck pain.

In closing this chapter, it's clear that exercises tailored to your neck's needs play a crucial role in maintaining health and preventing pain. From gentle movements to targeted strength-building routines, each exercise contributes to a stronger, more resilient neck. As you continue to explore these strategies, remember that consistency and mindfulness are your allies in achieving lasting relief. Looking forward, we'll explore how lifestyle adjustments and ergonomic changes can further enhance your path to a pain-free life.

4

POSTURE AND ALIGNMENT TECHNIQUES

Imagine stepping into a world where every movement exudes confidence and every stance reflects ease. This world is within reach when you embrace the power of proper posture. Good posture is more than standing tall; it is the alignment that supports your body's natural curves, reducing strain on your neck and spine. By understanding the fundamentals of posture, you unveil a path to comfort and agility, crucial for adults, athletes, and youth alike. Aligning your head correctly in relation to your shoulders and spine is the cornerstone of posture. This alignment minimizes the pressure on your cervical spine and prevents muscle overload, common issues in today's tech-driven society. Picture your head as a balanced sphere atop a tower; any forward tilt increases the tower's instability, placing undue strain on the neck and leading to the dreaded forward head posture.

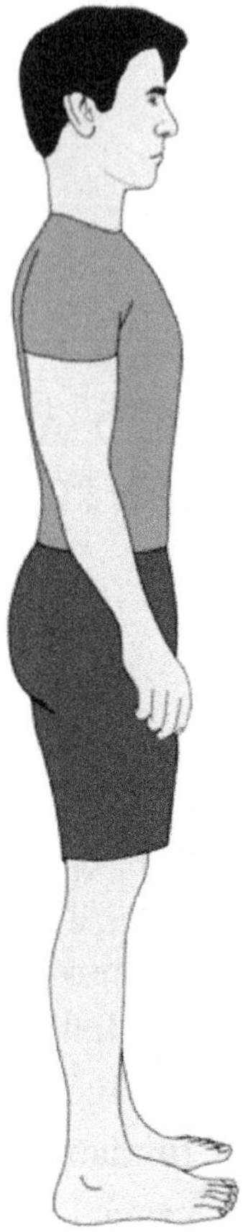

Fig 4.1 Neutral Spine

A neutral spine is your body's optimal alignment, maintaining the natural curve of your neck and lower back. This position distributes weight evenly, allowing your muscles and ligaments to function without undue stress. Whether you are sitting at a desk, running on a track, or standing in line, maintaining a neutral spine is essential. It supports your neck and enhances your overall posture, boosting confidence and reducing fatigue. Think of your spine as the central pillar of a building; its strength and alignment determine the structure's stability. By nurturing this alignment, you create a foundation that supports every movement with grace and efficiency.

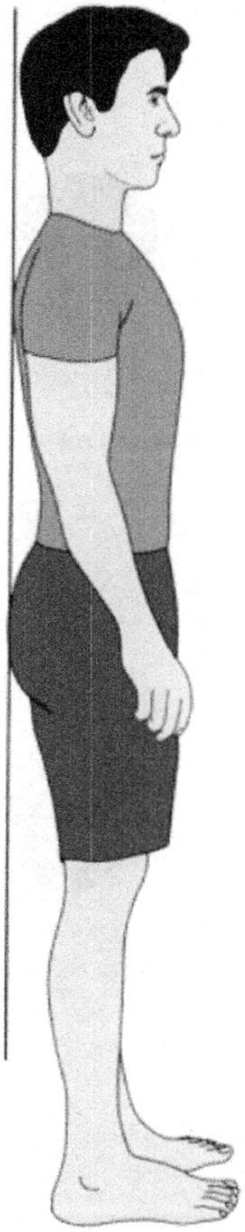

Fig 4.2 Wall Test

To cultivate good posture, integrate actionable correction techniques into your daily life. Begin with the wall test, a straightforward assessment of your posture. Stand with your back against a wall, ensuring that your head, shoulder blades, and buttocks touch the surface. The space between your lower back and the wall should be just enough for your hand to slide through. This position mirrors the neutral spine, revealing any deviations in your posture. By practicing this test regularly, you can develop a keen awareness of your alignment, guiding you toward better posture habits.

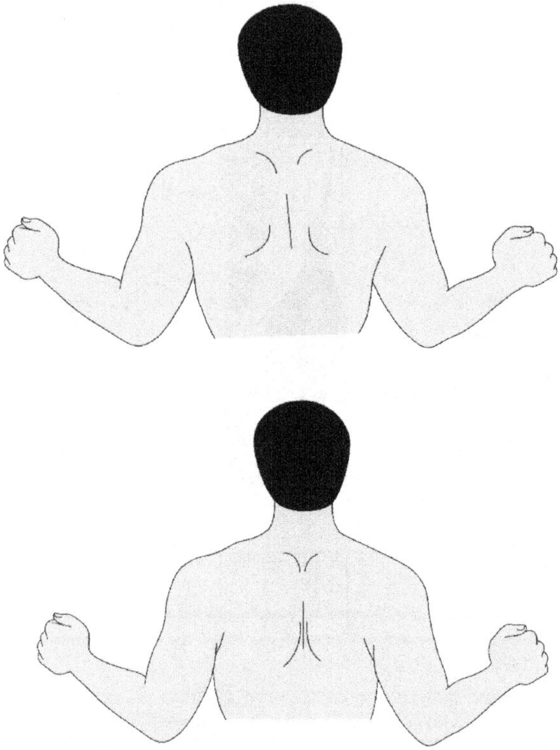

Fig 4.3 Shoulder Blade Retraction

Shoulder blade retraction exercises are another effective technique to counteract slumping. Stand or sit with your back straight and gently pull your shoulder blades together, as if attempting to hold a pencil between them. Hold this position for a few seconds before releasing. This exercise strengthens the muscles that support your upper back and neck, promoting improved alignment and reducing the tendency to slouch.

Common posture pitfalls can derail even the most diligent efforts. Slumping when sitting is a frequent mistake that leads to muscle fatigue and neck pain. This posture collapses the chest and rounds the shoulders, disrupting the neutral spine. To avoid slumping, ensure that your chair supports your lower back and that your feet rest flat on the floor. Adjust your desk and monitor height to encourage an upright position. Forward head posture, where the head juts forward beyond the shoulders, is another common issue. This position places significant strain on the cervical spine, increasing the risk of pain and degeneration. To combat this, regularly perform chin tucks and chest stretches, which realign the head over the shoulders and relax tight muscles.

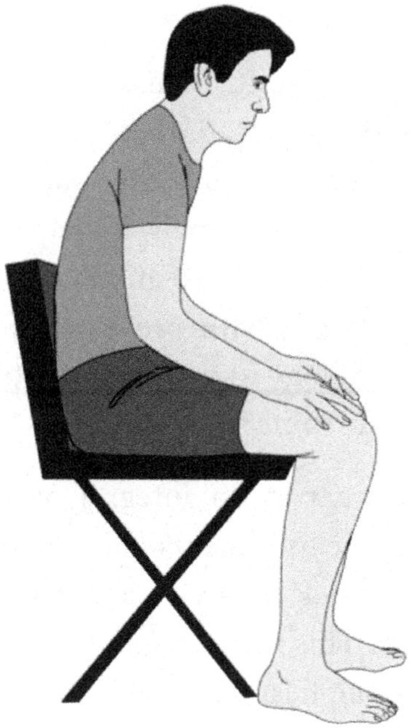

Fig 4.3 Slumping

Continuous self-awareness is the key to maintaining good posture. Develop a habit of checking your alignment throughout the day, whether at work, during exercise, or while relaxing. Set reminders to stand up, stretch, and reset your posture. Use visual cues, such as sticky notes or phone alerts, to prompt these checks, ensuring that posture correction becomes second nature. By fostering this mindfulness, you empower yourself to take control of your posture, enhancing your neck health and overall well-being. Embrace the journey toward better posture with patience and dedication, knowing that each adjustment brings you closer to a life free from neck pain and discomfort.

4.1 POSTURE CHECK 3D™ FROM FOOT LEVELERS

In our modern lives, where we are often glued to screens and seated for long stretches, maintaining proper posture has become a significant challenge. It's not just about aesthetics; poor posture can lead to a cascade of health issues, including persistent back pain, neck strain, and even headaches. The Posture Check 3D™ from Foot Levelers offers a cutting-edge solution to this pervasive problem, providing a detailed analysis that goes far beyond the superficial. Imagine being able to measure and understand the intricacies of your posture with precision. This innovative tool utilizes advanced technology to deliver insights that can transform how you approach your spine health.

The 3D Posture Scanner is an integral part of this system. It provides analytical measurements of forward head posture, known as the Tech Neck Index™, a condition exacerbated by prolonged device use. This measurement is crucial because even a slight forward tilt of the head can significantly increase the strain on the neck and upper back muscles. By understanding the degree of this posture deviation, you can take targeted steps to correct it, such as adjusting your workspace or incorporating specific exercises to strengthen the neck and shoulder muscles. The scanner's precision offers a clear picture of how your posture might be contributing to back pain and other discomforts, empowering you to make changes that have a real impact.

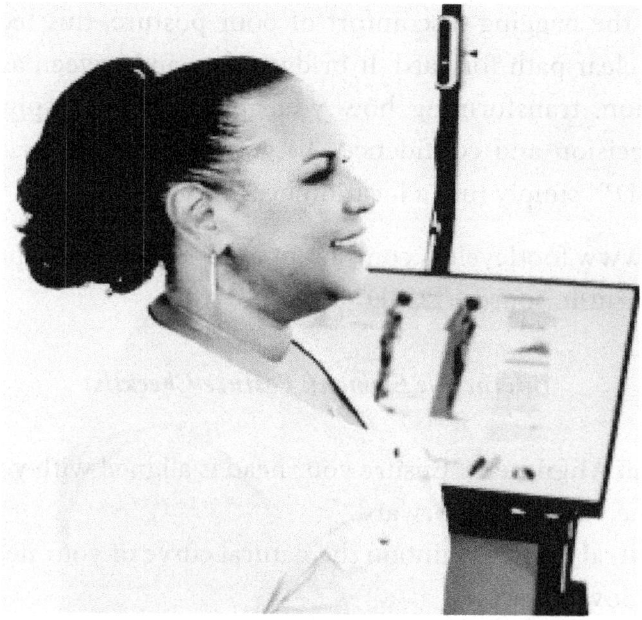

Fig 4.4 3D Posture Scanner

The Posture Check 3D™ system culminates in a Report of Findings, offering a full-body analysis from head to toe. This comprehensive report is not merely a collection of data points; it is a roadmap for improving your posture and, by extension, your overall health. By detailing where specific issues lie, the report helps you understand the interconnectedness of your body's alignment. With this knowledge, you can make informed decisions about your health, whether it's choosing to consult a specialist, adjusting your daily habits, or investing in supportive products.

For athletes, adults, and youth alike, the Posture Check 3D™ is a valuable tool in the quest for optimal health. It provides the insights needed to understand how posture affects your body, offering actionable data that can guide your efforts to improve alignment and reduce pain. Whether you're looking to enhance athletic performance, prevent future injuries, or simply live without the nagging discomfort of poor posture, this technology offers a clear path forward. It bridges the gap between awareness and action, transforming how you approach your spine health with precision and confidence. To get a complimentary Posture Check 3D™ simply find a location near you here:

https://www.footlevelers.com/about/find-a-healthcare-provider-near-you?utm_source=PC3D

Interactive Element: Posture Checklist

- **Head Alignment**: Ensure your head is aligned with your spine, not jutting forward.
- **Neutral Spine**: Maintain the natural curve of your neck and lower back.
- **Wall Test**: Stand against a wall to assess your posture.
- **Shoulder Blade Retraction**: Practice exercises to strengthen upper back muscles.
- **Awareness**: Regularly check and correct your posture throughout the day.

By incorporating these techniques, you pave the way for improved posture, reduced neck strain, and enhanced quality of life, regardless of age or activity level.

4.2 DESK JOCKEY SOLUTIONS: EXERCISES FOR OFFICE WORKERS

In the digital age, many find themselves shackled to a desk for hours on end, a reality that brings a unique set of challenges to posture and neck health. The sedentary nature of desk jobs significantly impacts posture, often leading to a cascade of musculoskeletal issues. When you sit for prolonged periods, your body tends to slouch, and your neck strains forward to meet the screen. This positioning can create an imbalance that exacerbates neck pain and stiffness. The constant gaze at computers or devices is a modern epidemic, contributing to what some call "tech neck," a condition that's as uncomfortable as it is preventable. This continuous cycle of poor posture leads to chronic tension in the neck and shoulders, further compounded by the lack of movement that comes with a sedentary lifestyle.

However, relief is within reach, and it starts right at your desk. Incorporating desk-friendly exercises into your routine can mitigate the adverse effects of prolonged sitting. Seated spinal twists are an excellent way to keep your spine flexible and relieve tension. Sit upright in your chair, feet flat on the floor. Place your right hand on the back of the chair and your left hand on your knee. Gently twist your torso to the right, feeling the stretch along your spine. Hold for a few breaths and then switch sides. This simple movement encourages mobility in the spine and can be performed discreetly throughout the day. Desk stretches for the neck and shoulders offer another layer of relief. Sit up straight and gently tilt your head towards one shoulder, holding for a few seconds before repeating on the opposite side. Follow this with a shoulder roll: lift your shoulders towards your ears, rotate them back, and then drop them down. These stretches can help release accumulated tension and promote better circulation in areas prone to stiffness from extended computer work.

To support these exercises, ergonomic adjustments at your workstation are crucial. An ergonomic chair with proper lumbar support can make a world of difference. Look for chairs that allow you to adjust the height, backrest angle, and armrests to suit your body. Your feet should rest comfortably on a footrest or flat on the floor to maintain a good posture. Position your computer monitor at eye level, about an arm's length away, to prevent you from craning your neck forward. This setup encourages a neutral head position, aligning your neck with your spine. Ergonomic keyboards and mouse devices also aid in reducing strain on the wrists and forearms, which can indirectly affect neck posture.

Beyond these tools, regular movement breaks are vital. These pauses are not merely a respite from work, but a necessary intervention to counteract the effects of sitting. Stand up and stretch every 30 minutes to an hour, allowing your body to reset. Walk around the office or perform light stretches that engage different muscle groups. These breaks enhance circulation, reduce fatigue, and provide a mental refresh, boosting productivity and maintaining focus. Consider setting a timer on your phone or computer as a reminder to take these mini-breaks, ensuring they become a consistent part of your workday routine. While the demands of desk work are undeniable, they need not doom you to a life of neck pain. By integrating these exercises and ergonomic practices into your daily routine, you protect your neck and shoulders from the rigors of modern office life. The goal is to create a dynamic work environment that supports your body, allowing you to perform at your best without compromising your health.

4.3 YOGA FOR NECK HEALTH: POSES TO ENHANCE FLEXIBILITY AND STRENGTH

Yoga stands as a beacon of relief for those suffering from neck tension and stiffness. Its benefits extend beyond the physical, touching on the mental and emotional realms, offering a holistic approach to health. When practiced consistently, yoga enhances flexibility, boosts strength, and improves alignment, all of which are crucial for maintaining neck health. The ancient art of yoga is particularly effective in reducing muscle tension, a common culprit behind neck discomfort. Through mindful movement and intentional stretching, yoga helps release tight muscles, promoting a state of relaxation that can be elusive in our fast-paced lives. The gentle, yet effective nature of yoga makes it accessible to everyone, regardless of age or fitness level, providing a pathway to greater physical harmony.

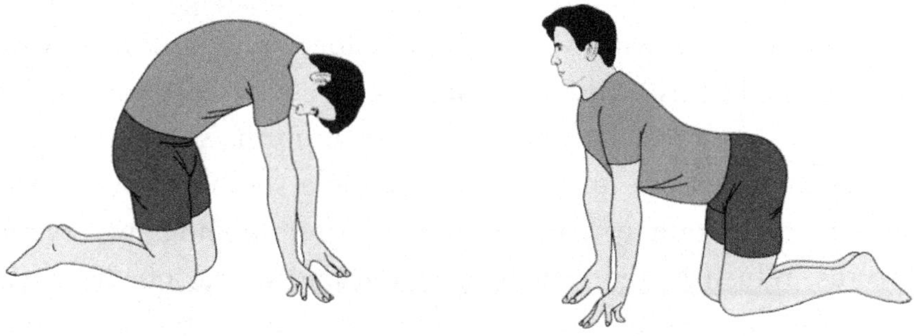

Fig 4.5 Cat - Cow Pose

A focal point of yoga's effectiveness lies in its ability to target specific areas like the neck and upper back. Take, for instance, the Cat-Cow pose, a staple in yoga practice known for its ability to increase spine flexibility and strength. This pose involves transitioning between two positions: the Cat pose, where the back is arched, and the Cow pose, where the back is concave. Start on all fours, aligning wrists under shoulders and knees under hips. Inhale as you drop your belly, lifting your head and tailbone for Cow pose; exhale as you round your back, tucking your chin to your chest for Cat pose. This rhythmic motion warms up the spine and releases tension in the neck, making it an excellent exercise for those seeking relief from stiffness.

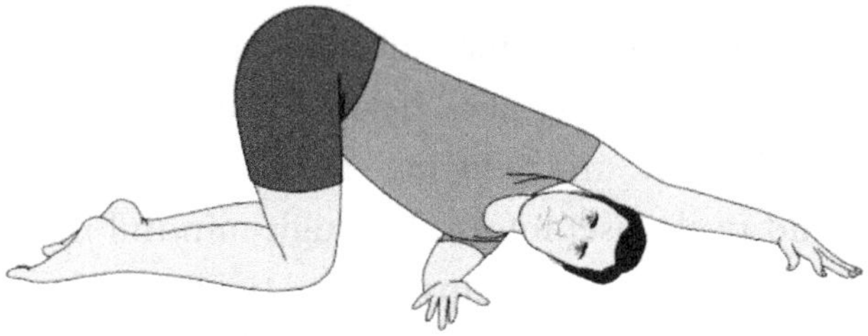

Fig 4.6 Thread the Needle

Another effective pose is Thread the Needle, which provides a deep stretch for the shoulders and neck. Begin on all fours, similar to the starting position of Cat-Cow. Slide your right arm under your left arm, allowing your right shoulder and cheek to rest on the mat. Hold this position, feeling the stretch across your upper back and shoulders. This pose helps open up the shoulder blades and releases tension in the neck, offering a soothing counterbalance to the strain of daily activities. After holding for several breaths, return to the starting position and repeat on the other side, ensuring that both sides of your body receive the benefits of this gentle stretch.

Breath work is integral to yoga, aiding in achieving deeper stretches and facilitating relaxation. The act of breathing deeply and consciously enhances the body's ability to stretch and helps maintain focus during each pose. Inhale deeply through the nose, allowing your ribcage to expand, and exhale slowly through the mouth, releasing any tension. This controlled breathing supports the physical execution of poses and calms the mind, reducing stress and its accompanying muscle tension. By integrating breath work into your practice, you cultivate a deeper connection between mind and body, enhancing the overall effectiveness of your yoga routine.

Yoga accommodates all levels, making it a versatile practice for anyone looking to improve neck health. For those new to yoga or experiencing limited flexibility, modifications can be made to ensure comfort and safety. Using props like blocks or straps can assist in achieving proper alignment and depth in poses. For example, if reaching the floor in Thread the Needle is challenging, place a block under your shoulder for support. These adaptations allow you to reap the benefits of yoga without strain, fostering a positive experience that encourages continued practice. More seasoned practitioners can explore deeper variations, enhancing the stretch and strengthening the muscles further.

4.4 PILATES FOR POSTURE: CORE EXERCISES TO SUPPORT YOUR NECK

Pilates offers a pathway to improved posture and neck alignment by focusing on core strength, a crucial element often overlooked in traditional exercise regimens. The core is not just about abdominal muscles; it includes the deep stabilizing muscles of the torso that support the spine's alignment. When these muscles are strong and engaged, they act like a natural corset, providing the foundation for a balanced and aligned body. This balance is vital for reducing neck strain, as a stable core prevents the upper body from compensating for weaknesses elsewhere. In essence, a strong core supports the spine like the roots of a tree, anchoring it firmly and allowing the branches—your limbs and head—to move freely without stress.

One of the cornerstone exercises in Pilates that exemplifies this core engagement is The Hundred. This exercise is designed to build endurance in the core muscles, promoting stability and strength. Begin by lying on your back with your legs raised to a tabletop position, knees bent at 90 degrees. Lift your head and shoulders off the mat, reaching your arms forward. Pump your arms up and down vigorously while inhaling for five counts and exhaling for five counts, completing a cycle of ten breaths. This rhythmic movement engages the core and encourages an awareness of your body's alignment, teaching you to maintain stability even under dynamic conditions. The Hundred is a testament to how core exercises in Pilates can support neck health by reinforcing the body's central pillar.

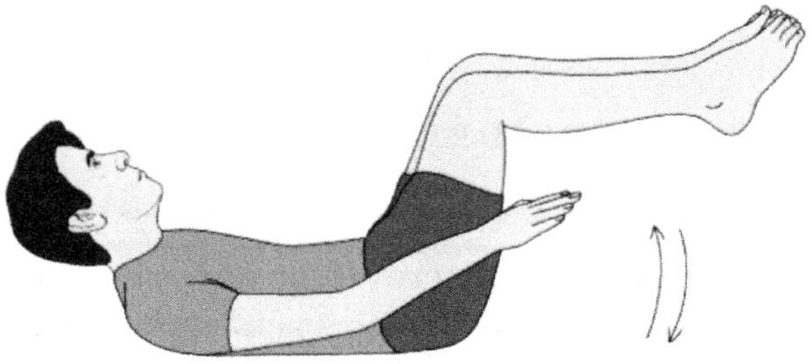

Fig 4.6 The Hundred

The connection between core strength and neck health cannot be overstated. A robust core acts as a stabilizing force, preventing the upper body from collapsing or compensating with poor posture. This stability reduces the load on the neck, which can otherwise become a site of tension and discomfort. When the core is weak, the neck often bears the brunt of maintaining balance and alignment, leading to strain and potential injury. By fortifying the core through Pilates, you provide a solid foundation that alleviates pressure on the neck and promotes overall body symmetry.

Maintaining proper form and technique is paramount in Pilates, where precision takes precedence over speed or repetition. Ensure that movements are controlled and deliberate, focusing on the quality of each exercise rather than the quantity. Engage the core consistently, using your breath to enhance movement precision and control. Keep the neck relaxed, avoiding unnecessary tension, and maintain an awareness of your body's alignment throughout each exercise. This attention to detail not only maximizes the benefits of Pilates for posture and neck support but also minimizes the risk of injury. Proper form ensures that you target the right muscles, reinforcing the connection between core strength and neck health effectively.

4.5 THE ROLE OF ALIGNMENT IN NECK HEALTH: UNDERSTANDING BODY MECHANICS

The concept of body mechanics is often overlooked, yet it plays a pivotal role in maintaining neck health and overall physical well-being. Body mechanics refers to the way we move our bodies, ensuring that alignment is maintained during all activities. Proper alignment minimizes stress and strain on the neck and spine, reducing the risk of injuries and chronic pain. Imagine your body as a finely tuned machine, where each part must work harmoniously with the others to function optimally. When the hips, spine, and head are correctly aligned, the body operates efficiently, distributing forces evenly and preventing undue stress on any one area.

Consider the simple act of lifting an object. Proper lifting techniques are crucial to avoiding neck strain. Always bend at the knees and hips, rather than the waist, keeping your back straight.

Hold the object close to your body and lift with your legs, not your back. This method ensures that the load is distributed through the stronger muscles of the lower body, protecting the neck and spine from excessive strain. Similarly, alignment during walking and running is vital. Ensure that your head is held high, shoulders are back, and core is engaged. This posture promotes better breathing and oxygenation and alleviates stress on the neck, allowing for smoother and more efficient movement.

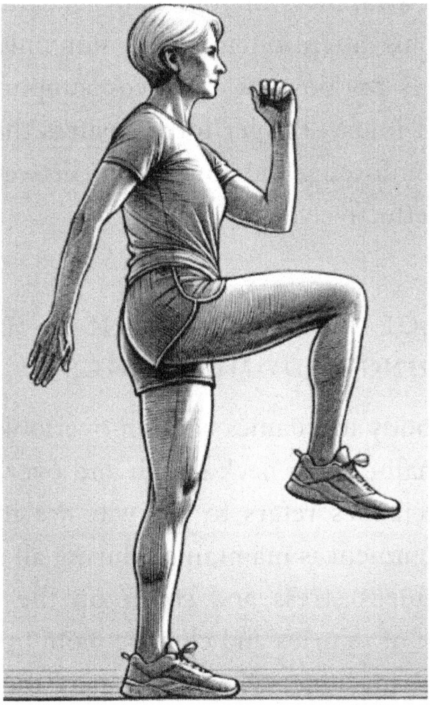

Fig 4.7 One Leg Standing Balance

To improve body mechanics, incorporate exercises that enhance awareness and control over your movements. Balancing exercises are particularly effective for developing stability and coordination. Simple exercises, such as standing on one foot or using a balance board, challenge your body's ability to maintain equilibrium.

These activities engage the core and stabilizing muscles, reinforcing proper alignment during dynamic movements. As you gain proficiency, incorporate more complex movements that mimic daily activities, such as reaching or twisting, to further enhance your body's coordination and control.

While many individuals can make significant progress on their own, seeking professional guidance can provide a personalized approach to improving body mechanics. Physical therapists specialize in assessing and correcting alignment issues, offering tailored exercises and adjustments that address your specific needs. They can identify subtle misalignments and provide feedback on proper form and technique, ensuring that you maximize the benefits of your efforts. Consulting with a physical therapist can be especially beneficial if you have a history of injuries or chronic pain, as they can develop a comprehensive plan that promotes healing and prevents future issues.

Understanding and applying the principles of body mechanics is a continuous process, one that requires awareness and practice in every aspect of life. By focusing on alignment and movement, you empower yourself to maintain a healthy neck and spine, enhancing your ability to perform both daily tasks and athletic pursuits with ease.

4.6 VISUALIZING SUCCESS: USING IMAGERY TO ENHANCE POSTURE AND REDUCE PAIN

Visualization is an often-overlooked tool in the quest for better posture and reduced neck pain. It harnesses the power of your mind to create physical change, a technique widely used by athletes to enhance performance. Imagine a string gently pulling your head upwards, elongating your spine and aligning your head perfectly over your shoulders. This mental image helps correct posture naturally, encouraging you to stand taller and more confidently. Visualization is not just about imagining perfection; it's about creating a mental blueprint that guides your body into healthier patterns.

To effectively use visualization, begin by closing your eyes and picturing your shoulder blades gliding smoothly down your back. This imagery encourages the muscles to relax, reducing tension in the neck and upper back. Visualizing this movement can help correct slumping, a common issue for many. When you focus on this mental picture, your body responds, subtly adjusting to the visual cue. It's as if the mind and body are in a dance, with the brain leading and the body following rhythmically. This technique can be practiced anywhere, whether sitting at a desk or waiting in line, making it a versatile tool for posture correction.

Beyond physical alignment, visualization offers profound psychological benefits. It can enhance motivation and confidence, two crucial components in maintaining good posture. When you visualize success, you set a positive tone for your actions, encouraging consistency in your efforts. This mental rehearsal prepares you to face challenges with a sense of readiness and optimism. Visualization acts as a mental rehearsal, boosting your confidence in your body's ability to achieve and maintain proper posture. The mind-body connection is powerful, and by engaging in visualization, you strengthen this link, reinforcing positive habits and reducing neck discomfort over time.

Consider the story of Jordan, a young professional who struggled with persistent neck pain due to long hours at a computer. Traditional methods offered limited relief, but visualization transformed his approach. By spending a few moments each morning imagining his posture as a strong, supportive framework, Jordan noticed a significant decrease in neck tension. His confidence grew as he felt more in control of his body's alignment, and he carried this newfound awareness into his daily activities. Visualization became a cornerstone of his routine, guiding him toward lasting improvement.

Visualization is accessible to everyone, regardless of age or physical ability, and offers a unique way to engage the mind in the pursuit of physical health. It empowers you to take an active role in your well-being, providing a sense of agency in managing neck pain. This practice encourages mindfulness, fostering a deeper awareness of your body's signals and needs. As you incorporate visualization into your daily life, remember that it's a journey, not a destination. Consistency is key, and over time, you'll find that this mental exercise corrects posture and enriches your overall sense of well-being. Visualization opens a door to a new dimension of self-care, where the mind and body collaborate to create a state of balance and harmony.

With visualization as a powerful ally, you can approach posture correction and pain reduction with renewed vigor and insight. This chapter has explored the various techniques and strategies to support neck health through posture and alignment. As you move forward, consider how these practices can be integrated into a holistic approach to well-being, setting the stage for the next chapter where we delve into lifestyle changes that complement these physical adjustments, creating a comprehensive strategy for neck health.

BETTER THAN PAINKILLERS

"Take care of your body. It's the only place you have to live."

— *JIM ROHN*

As you may remember, up to 70% of adults will experience neck pain at some point. When I was a practicing sports chiropractor, teaching people how to manage and relieve pain was a common task, and while I have no problem with painkillers, I would never have suggested that anyone rely on them solely. For many people, though, this is the reality. They don't realize how much they can do with exercise and lifestyle changes—things that are so powerful that, when incorporated into regular life, often do away with the need for painkillers entirely. What happens is that people numb the pain during the moments when it's unbearable, and then the underlying causes persist, and the cycle begins again.

When I retired, I realized I wasn't ready to let all my work go. I wanted to continue to help people, and I wanted to reach more people than I'd ever be able to see in my practice. Neck pain can be debilitating, and if I can help just a fraction of the 70% of adults who experience it, I'll be happy.

I know you understand how much of a problem neck pain can be; if you didn't, you wouldn't be reading this book. If you're finding what you're learning here helpful, it would be wonderful if you could take a moment to help more people who are suffering from neck pain to find it and learn what they can do to find relief. The only thing you have to do to make that happen is to leave a short review.

By leaving a review of this book on Amazon, you'll make it more visible when people are searching for solutions to neck pain, and they'll be able to equip themselves with these strategies.

There are a lot of people out there suffering from neck pain because modern life requires us to put a lot of strain on our necks. But we can do something about this, and by helping me get this book to more of the people who need it, you could make a huge difference in someone else's life.

Thank you for your support. I truly appreciate it.

Scan the QR code below:

5

PAIN MANAGEMENT AND QUICK RELIEF STRATEGIES

Imagine a day where you're fully engaged in activities, only to be interrupted by the familiar twinge of neck tension. It's a discomfort many know too well, often creeping up unexpectedly, demanding immediate attention. Fortunately, several instant relief techniques can provide the reprieve you need to continue your day uninterrupted. These methods, when incorporated into your routine, can offer a powerful defense against the persistent nuisance of neck pain.

Neck stretches are a cornerstone of instant relief, offering a simple yet effective way to release tension. Begin with the forward and backward tilt, where you stand or sit with your head aligned over your shoulders. Lower your chin gently towards your chest, holding the position for 15 to 30 seconds, breathing deeply to enhance the stretch. Once complete, tilt your head back and gaze upward, holding again for a few seconds. This movement alleviates stiffness and restores flexibility, making it ideal for those moments when your neck feels particularly tight. Side tilts complement this routine by targeting lateral tension. With your feet hip-width apart, tilt your head towards one shoulder, hold the stretch, and repeat on the opposite side. These exercises, simple yet impactful, can be seamlessly integrated into your day, providing a quick path to relaxation.

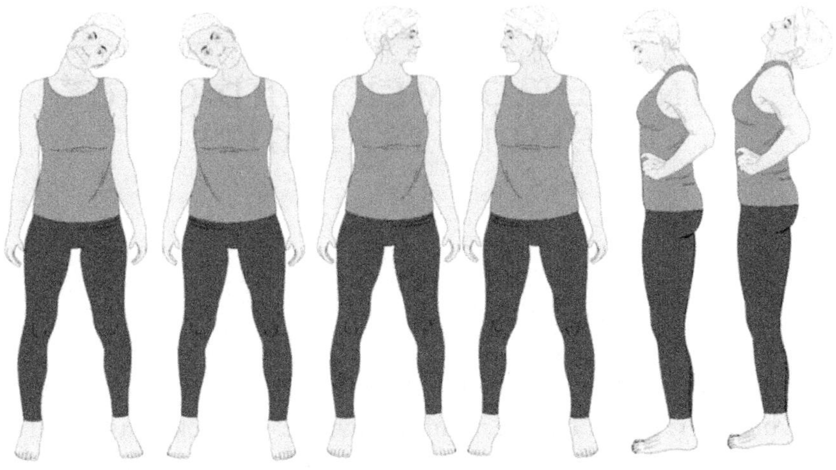

Fig 5.1 Neck Stretching

Acupressure offers another layer of relief by tapping into the body's meridian points to alleviate pain. The Wind Pool, located at the base of the skull behind the earlobe, is particularly effective for neck tension. Applying gentle pressure in a circular motion for a few minutes can soothe muscles and improve circulation, reducing discomfort. Another point, Heaven's Pillar, is found on either side of the neck. Massaging these areas can relieve congestion and tension, offering a holistic approach to neck pain management. Incorporating acupressure into your routine provides a natural and accessible way to combat pain, with the added benefit of promoting overall relaxation.

Mobility exercises further enhance neck health by keeping muscles active and joints supple. Neck rotations, for example, increase blood flow and maintain flexibility. Stand or sit comfortably, and gently rotate your head from side to side, pausing at each end of the movement. This exercise reduces tension and improves your range of motion, essential for maintaining a healthy neck. Performing these rotations regularly prevents stiffness, especially after prolonged periods of inactivity, such as sitting at a desk or during long commutes.

Sometimes, over-the-counter aids can offer additional support in managing neck pain. Topical analgesics, available in creams or gels, provide targeted relief by numbing the area and reducing inflammation. These products are easy to apply and act quickly, offering a soothing sensation that can alleviate discomfort. Keep a small tube or bottle handy at home or in your gym bag, ready to use when tension strikes unexpectedly. The convenience of these aids makes them a practical addition to your pain management toolkit, complementing stretches and exercises for a well-rounded approach to relief.

Consistency in practicing these techniques is key to preventing neck pain from becoming a recurring issue. By incorporating stretches, acupressure, and mobility exercises into your daily routine, you create a proactive strategy for maintaining neck health. Set aside a few moments each day, whether during a work break or at the start of your morning routine, to perform these exercises. This regular practice provides immediate relief and strengthens your neck over time, reducing the likelihood of future pain. Embracing these techniques as part of your lifestyle empowers you to take control of your neck health, enabling you to live with less pain and more freedom.

5.1 HEAT AND COLD THERAPY: WHEN AND HOW TO USE THEM

Navigating the landscape of neck pain relief often brings you to the twin pillars of heat and cold therapy. These methods, rooted in ancient practices yet supported by modern science, offer distinct benefits for managing discomfort. Heat therapy, for instance, invites relaxation by dilating blood vessels, which increases circulation and delivers essential nutrients to muscles. This warmth penetrates deeply, easing tightness and promoting flexibility. Imagine wrapping a warm towel around your neck on a chilly evening, feeling the soothing embrace as tension slowly melts away. Heat is particularly beneficial for chronic neck pain, where muscle stiffness persists long after the initial injury has healed. By applying heat, you encourage the muscles to relax, allowing for greater freedom of movement.

In contrast, cold therapy serves as a defender against swelling and acute pain. It works by constricting blood vessels, reducing circulation to the affected area, which helps numb pain and minimize inflammation. Picture an athlete applying an ice pack to a fresh injury, feeling the immediate cooling relief as the cold numbs the throbbing ache. This method is ideal for recent neck injuries or flare-ups, where reducing swelling is paramount. The cold acts as a natural analgesic, dulling pain signals and providing quick, albeit temporary, relief. By understanding these fundamental principles, you can make informed decisions about which therapy to use based on the nature of your neck pain.

To safely and effectively apply these therapies, certain guidelines must be followed. For heat therapy, a heating pad or warm towel is often the most accessible option. Ensure the temperature is comfortable—not too hot to avoid burns—and apply it to the neck for 15 to 20 minutes at a time. This duration allows the heat to penetrate without causing overheating. If using a towel, dampen it slightly before warming it in a microwave, then wrap it around your neck for a cozy, spa-like experience. Cold therapy typically involves an ice pack wrapped in a thin cloth to protect the skin. Apply it to the painful area for 15 to 20 minutes, allowing the cold to soothe inflammation. Repeat this process every few hours as needed, but always give your skin time to warm up between applications to prevent frostbite.

Timing and frequency are crucial when employing heat and cold therapy. For acute injuries, prioritize cold treatments during the first 48 hours to control swelling and manage pain. As the initial inflammation subsides, transition to heat therapy to relax muscles and improve mobility. For chronic neck pain, heat therapy can be used regularly to maintain muscle flexibility and reduce persistent tension. Alternating between hot and cold treatments, known as contrast therapy, can also be effective, as it stimulates circulation and accelerates healing. However, it's important to use these therapies judiciously, as overuse can lead to skin irritation or exacerbate your symptoms.

Finally, while heat and cold therapies are generally safe, they are not without risks. Avoid applying heat to an acute injury, as it can increase swelling and prolong recovery. Similarly, refrain from using cold packs directly on the skin or for extended periods, as this can cause frostbite. Always listen to your body and adjust the temperature and duration according to your comfort level. If you experience any adverse reactions, discontinue use and consult a healthcare professional. By respecting these precautionary measures, you ensure that heat and cold therapies remain valuable tools in your neck pain management arsenal.

5.2 TRIGGER POINT THERAPY: SELF-MASSAGE TECHNIQUES FOR PAIN RELIEF

In the intricate web of muscle fibers that make up your neck and shoulders, certain spots can become sources of pain and discomfort. These are known as myofascial trigger points. Think of them as knots in a rope, areas where muscle fibers have tightened and contracted, often due to stress, poor posture, or overuse. These trigger points can refer pain to other parts of your neck and even lead to headaches. Understanding how to address them through self-massage can be a game changer in managing chronic neck tension.

When it comes to self-massage for trigger points, the process is straightforward yet requires attention to detail. Begin by locating the area of discomfort. Often, trigger points will feel like small, tender nodules within the muscle. Use your fingers to apply firm, steady pressure directly onto the knot. This pressure should be deep enough to reach the underlying muscle, but not so intense that it causes sharp pain. If you prefer, massage tools such as a tennis ball or a specialized massage roller can help reach deeper points, especially in hard-to-reach areas like between the shoulder blades.

For the neck and shoulder areas, a simple yet effective technique involves using your thumb and forefinger to pinch the muscle between them. Gently roll the muscle between your fingers, applying consistent pressure. This can help release tension and improve circulation, aiding in the muscle's return to a relaxed state. For the upper trapezius muscles, which often bear the brunt of stress, use a cross-fiber massage technique. Place your fingers on the muscle and move them side to side, perpendicular to the muscle fibers, which helps break down adhesions and ease stiffness.

Regular practice of trigger point therapy can significantly reduce tension and improve mobility. By incorporating these techniques into your weekly routine, you can alleviate discomfort before it escalates into more severe pain. This proactive approach helps maintain muscle flexibility and resilience, allowing you to move with greater ease and confidence. It's a simple yet effective way to take control of your neck health, offering relief and freedom from the constraints of chronic pain.

As with any self-care practice, caution is essential. Always listen to your body's signals and respect its limits. If you encounter a trigger point that remains stubbornly painful despite self-massage, or if the discomfort spreads or intensifies, it may be time to consult a healthcare professional. A physical therapist or massage therapist can provide a more comprehensive assessment and offer targeted treatments that address the underlying causes of your pain. Remember, while self-massage is a valuable tool, it is not a substitute for professional medical advice or intervention.

5.3 BREATHING EXERCISES FOR STRESS-INDUCED NECK PAIN

The connection between stress and neck pain is undeniable, often manifesting as tightness and discomfort that can be both persistent and debilitating. At the heart of this relationship is the role of stress in triggering muscle tension, particularly in the neck and shoulders. Fortunately, breathing exercises offer a natural and effective way to alleviate this tension. By engaging in deep diaphragmatic breathing, you can activate the body's relaxation response, which counteracts the effects of stress hormones. This method involves inhaling deeply through your nose, allowing your diaphragm to expand fully, then exhaling slowly and completely through your mouth. This type of breathing encourages a calmer state of mind, which translates into physical relaxation, easing the tightness in your neck.

One specific technique that can be particularly beneficial is box breathing. This exercise is known for its calming effects and simplicity. To practice box breathing, sit comfortably and inhale slowly through your nose for a count of four. Hold your breath for another count of four, then exhale slowly through your mouth for four counts. Finally, pause and hold your breath again for four counts before repeating the cycle. This structured pattern not only helps stabilize your breathing but also instills a sense of control and calm, which can markedly decrease neck tension. The rhythmic nature of box breathing promotes a meditative state, providing an especially useful mental and physical reset in high-stress situations.

Another effective exercise is alternate nostril breathing, which is traditionally used in yoga for balancing the body's energy. This technique involves closing one nostril with your thumb and inhaling deeply through the other. After holding the breath briefly, switch nostrils by closing the one you inhaled through and exhaling through the opposite side. Continue alternating in this manner, focusing on the steady flow of your breath. This exercise not only balances your breathing but also enhances mental clarity and reduces stress, contributing to a reduction in neck tension. The emphasis on controlled, mindful breathing encourages a slower heart rate and a calm mind, both of which are conducive to alleviating muscle tightness.

The benefits of regular practice of these breathing exercises extend beyond immediate stress relief. Consistent engagement with these techniques can lead to improved overall well-being, as they foster a sense of mindfulness and presence. Over time, you may notice a general decrease in stress levels, improved focus, and a greater capacity to handle stressful situations without physical repercussions. By incorporating these exercises into your daily routine, you create a buffer against the stressors that contribute to neck pain, enhancing both mental and physical health. This regular practice becomes a cornerstone of a balanced lifestyle, promoting resilience and well-being.

Creating a conducive environment for breathing exercises is key to maximizing their effectiveness. Choose a quiet, comfortable space where you can sit or lie down without disturbances. Early morning or before bedtime are particularly good times for practice when your mind is naturally more receptive to relaxation techniques. Dim lighting, soft music, or natural sounds can enhance the calming atmosphere, allowing you to focus entirely on your breathing. By setting aside dedicated time for these exercises, you establish a routine that prioritizes self-care and relaxation. This intentional practice addresses neck pain and nurtures a holistic approach to stress management, contributing to a healthier, more balanced life.

5.4 IDENTIFYING AND AVOIDING EXERCISE MISTAKES THAT AGGRAVATE PAIN

Embarking on an exercise regimen can be both exhilarating and intimidating, especially when dealing with neck pain. While the benefits of staying active are well-documented, certain exercise mistakes can inadvertently exacerbate neck pain. A prime culprit is incorrect form during weightlifting. Many individuals, keen to see quick results, may rush through their sets, neglecting the importance of alignment. When lifting weights, it's crucial to maintain a neutral spine, keeping the head aligned with the torso. Allowing the neck to jut forward or overextending can place undue stress on cervical vertebrae, leading to discomfort or injury. Overstretching, another common error, can also lead to muscle strain. While stretching is integral to maintaining flexibility, pushing beyond your limits can cause the muscles to tighten reflexively, increasing the risk of injury. It's essential to listen to your body's cues and respect its current range of motion.

Corrective measures are vital to ensure that your exercise routine supports rather than hinders your neck health. Begin by focusing on proper alignment, which serves as the foundation for all exercises. Whether you're lifting weights or performing yoga, always be mindful of your posture. Engage your core muscles to support your spine, and keep your head aligned with your body. Controlled movements are equally important. Rather than prioritizing speed, concentrate on the quality of each rep or stretch. This approach minimizes the risk of injury and ensures that you engage the correct muscle groups. For instance, when performing a shoulder press, move slowly and deliberately, feeling the muscles work with each lift. This heightened awareness transforms each session into an opportunity to refine your technique and strengthen your body safely.

Listening to your body is another critical aspect of effective exercise. Pain is a signal that something is amiss, and ignoring it can have long-term consequences. If you experience discomfort during a particular movement, pause and assess your form. It may be necessary to modify the exercise or reduce the intensity. For example, if a particular weight feels too heavy, don't hesitate to lighten the load. Pushing through pain is never advisable and can lead to more severe issues down the line. Instead, approach each workout with patience, recognizing that progress is a marathon, not a sprint. By tuning into your body's signals, you can tailor your routine to your needs, ensuring that it remains beneficial and sustainable.

When in doubt, consulting a professional can provide invaluable guidance. A physical therapist or certified trainer can assess your form and offer personalized advice to optimize your routine. These experts can identify subtle errors you might overlook and suggest modifications to enhance your performance and safety. They can also introduce exercises specifically designed to strengthen the neck and surrounding muscles, further reducing the risk of pain. Consider scheduling a session with a professional if you're new to exercise or have specific concerns about neck pain. Their insights can empower you to approach your fitness journey with confidence and clarity.

5.5 EMERGENCY PAIN STRATEGIES: WHAT TO DO WHEN PAIN STRIKES

In the realm of neck pain, emergencies can catch you off guard, demanding immediate attention. Recognizing when a situation qualifies as an emergency is crucial. A sudden onset of severe pain or a loss of mobility can feel alarming, and rightly so. These symptoms might indicate a more serious underlying issue, such as a nerve impingement or a disc herniation. When you experience such intense pain, it's important to act swiftly to prevent further complications. This is not the time to push through or ignore symptoms, as doing so could exacerbate the condition. Understanding that these situations require prompt action can make all the difference in recovery.

When faced with acute neck pain, having a plan can provide both physical relief and peace of mind. Begin by resting and immobilizing your neck. Find a comfortable position, perhaps reclining with pillows supporting your head and neck to minimize movement. This rest helps reduce strain on the affected area, allowing muscles to relax. Applying cold therapy can also be beneficial in the first 24 to 48 hours. Use an ice pack wrapped in a cloth to reduce inflammation and numb the pain, applying it for 15 to 20 minutes at a time. This approach can help manage swelling and provide temporary relief from the intense discomfort. Remember, these steps are meant to stabilize the situation and should be followed by a more comprehensive assessment if symptoms persist.

Recognizing when to seek medical attention is a critical component of managing neck pain effectively. If your pain does not improve with home strategies, or if it intensifies, it's wise to consult a healthcare professional. Persistent pain, particularly when accompanied by numbness, tingling, or weakness in the arms or legs, warrants further investigation. These symptoms might suggest nerve involvement, which requires a thorough evaluation to determine the best course of treatment. Consulting with a doctor ensures that you receive a proper diagnosis and tailored treatment plan, reducing the risk of long-term complications.

During these challenging moments, reassurance and coping strategies can help you stay calm. Remember that acute pain episodes, although distressing, are often manageable with the right approach. Deep breathing exercises can help alleviate anxiety, providing a moment of calm amidst the discomfort. Focus on slow, steady breaths to reduce stress levels and encourage relaxation. Visualization techniques, where you picture the pain subsiding and your muscles relaxing, can also be beneficial. Engaging in these mental exercises can distract from the pain, fostering a sense of control over the situation.

Having a checklist of emergency steps handy can empower you to act decisively. This list serves as a guide, ensuring that you don't overlook crucial steps in the heat of the moment. By preparing in advance, you can face sudden neck pain with confidence, knowing that you have a strategy in place. Empowerment comes from knowledge, and in these situations, being informed about potential actions can transform a daunting experience into a manageable one.

By understanding and implementing these emergency pain strategies, you equip yourself with tools to navigate acute neck pain effectively. This proactive approach addresses immediate symptoms and lays the groundwork for long-term management and recovery.

As we move forward in this guide, we'll explore how lifestyle adaptations can further mitigate neck pain, creating a comprehensive framework for sustained relief.

6

INTEGRATING MENTAL WELLNESS AND NECK HEALTH

Picture yourself in a moment of profound stress, where the weight of the world seems to rest squarely on your shoulders. In such times, it's not uncommon to feel that tension manifest physically, particularly as a knot in your neck. This is the mind-body connection in action. Mental health issues like stress and anxiety don't just reside in your mind; they often migrate, settling into your muscles and joints. Stress can cause your muscles to tense and contract, especially those in your neck and shoulders. This tension is a natural response to perceived threats, a remnant of our evolutionary past when such alertness might have saved us from danger.

The physiological link between mental health and physical symptoms like neck pain is significant. When you're stressed or anxious, your body activates the fight-or-flight response, an ancient survival mechanism designed to prepare you for immediate action. This response floods your system with stress hormones, increasing heart rate and muscle tension. While this is beneficial in life-threatening situations, in today's world, such responses are often triggered by non-physical threats like deadlines, exams, or personal conflicts. The result is chronic muscle tension, particularly in your neck, where the weight of stress physically settles.

Anxiety doesn't only affect muscle tension; it also impacts posture. When anxious, you might unconsciously hunch your shoulders or lower your head, contributing to poor posture. Over time, these subtle adjustments become habitual, exacerbating neck pain. The cycle is self-perpetuating: anxiety leads to poor posture, which causes neck pain, which in turn heightens anxiety. Addressing both the mental and physical aspects of this cycle is crucial for effective relief.

The nervous system plays a pivotal role in how mental states affect physical health. It serves as the communication network between your mind and body, translating mental states into physical responses. Consider the fight-or-flight response: as stress signals flood your body, the nervous system ramps up muscle tension and alertness, preparing you to react. However, when these signals persist, they lead to chronic tension, particularly in the neck and shoulders, areas already prone to stress accumulation. This constant state of readiness drains energy and heightens pain perception, making even minor discomfort feel overwhelming.

Real-life examples illustrate the profound impact of mental health on neck pain. Take Sarah, a college student whose academic pressures led to persistent neck stiffness. Her anxiety about exams caused her to spend hours hunched over textbooks, unaware of her tense posture. Over time, her neck pain became a constant companion, interfering with her studies and sleep. However, once she began addressing her anxiety through counseling and relaxation techniques, Sarah noticed a significant reduction in her neck pain. Her story underscores the importance of treating mental health issues to alleviate physical symptoms.

The importance of mental well-being in managing neck pain cannot be overstated. A balanced approach that considers both mental and physical health is vital for effective pain management. By nurturing mental wellness, you can reduce the stress and anxiety that contribute to muscle tension and poor posture. Techniques like relaxation exercises, counseling, and stress management strategies are valuable tools in this endeavor. By creating a supportive environment for mental health, you lay the foundation for physical relief.

Interactive Element: A Reflection on Stress Triggers

Consider taking a moment to reflect on your personal stress triggers. Use a journal to note situations or thoughts that consistently lead to tension. Identify patterns that link mental states to physical symptoms. This exercise can provide insight into how your mental health affects your neck, empowering you to develop strategies for relief.

6.1 MEDITATION PRACTICES FOR PAIN REDUCTION AND RELAXATION

Meditation stands as an invaluable tool in the realm of pain management, offering a path to alleviate stress and, consequently, neck pain. At the heart of meditation lies mindfulness, a practice of cultivating awareness of the present moment. This awareness extends to your body, fostering an understanding of how stress manifests physically. When stress grips you, it often tightens your neck and shoulders, creating a cycle of tension and pain. Through mindfulness meditation, you can gently guide your attention to these areas, acknowledging the tension and inviting relaxation. This practice encourages you to observe your sensations without judgment, allowing your mind and body to settle into a state of calm.

Guided imagery is another meditation technique that can profoundly impact your ability to manage pain. By engaging your imagination, you can visualize serene landscapes or comforting scenarios, easing mental stress and promoting physical relaxation. This imagery acts as a refuge, a place where your mind can retreat from the chaos of daily life. To practice guided imagery, find a quiet space where you can sit or lie comfortably. Close your eyes and take slow, deep breaths. Picture a scene that brings you peace —a tranquil beach, a lush forest, or a quiet meadow. Immerse yourself in the details: the sound of waves, the rustle of leaves, the warmth of the sun. This imagery helps your mind unwind, reducing the tension in your neck and shoulders.

The body scan meditation further aids in identifying and releasing tension. This practice involves systematically focusing on different parts of your body, fostering a deeper connection with your physical self. Begin by lying down in a comfortable position. Close your eyes and focus on your breathing, allowing it to become slow and steady. Start with your toes, noticing any sensations present, and gradually move your attention upward through your feet, legs, torso, arms, neck, and head. As you scan each area, observe any tension or discomfort without attempting to change it. Acknowledge these sensations with a sense of curiosity, and with each exhale, imagine the tension dissolving away. This meditation not only eases physical strain but also enhances your awareness of the connection between your mind and body.

Regular meditation practice yields significant benefits, extending far beyond immediate relaxation. Consistency is key, as the cumulative effect of meditation enhances your ability to manage stress and regulate emotions. Over time, you'll find yourself better equipped to handle the challenges that life presents. This improved emotional regulation can lead to sustained pain relief, as your body becomes less reactive to stressors. Meditation also encourages a more balanced approach to life's demands, fostering resilience and promoting overall well-being. As you integrate meditation into your routine, you may notice a heightened sense of clarity and focus, attributes that further support your journey towards neck pain relief.

For beginners, starting a meditation practice may seem daunting, but with a few simple steps, you can ease into it. Begin by setting aside a regular time each day, even if it's just five minutes, to practice meditation. Consistency is more important than duration, as it helps establish a habit. Create a space in your home that feels peaceful and free from distractions. This could be a corner of a room with a cushion or chair where you can sit comfortably. Remember, meditation is a personal practice, and it's essential to approach it without judgment or expectation. Allow yourself the freedom to explore different techniques, finding what resonates with you.

As you embrace meditation, you'll find it becomes a valuable ally in managing neck pain. The practice encourages a shift from tension to relaxation, from stress to peace. By dedicating time to meditation, you nurture your mind and body, paving the way for healing and relief.

6.2 COGNITIVE BEHAVIORAL STRATEGIES FOR MANAGING PAIN

Cognitive Behavioral Therapy, or CBT, offers a structured yet flexible framework to address the way you perceive and react to pain. At its core, CBT is about identifying and reshaping the negative thought patterns that often surround chronic pain. These thoughts can be insidious, quietly influencing how you feel and respond to discomfort. For instance, you might catch yourself thinking, "This pain will never get better," or, "I can't do anything because of my neck." These thoughts magnify the pain and limit your ability to cope effectively. By reframing these thoughts into more positive, realistic ones, you can reduce the pain's perceived intensity and impact on your life. CBT encourages you to develop positive coping strategies, fostering resilience and a more proactive approach to managing your discomfort. This shift in perspective can empower you to regain control over your pain, leading to a more balanced, less stressful experience.

To actively engage with CBT, you can use specific exercises designed to challenge and change your thoughts. One practical tool is the thought record worksheet, a simple yet powerful exercise that helps you dissect and understand the nature of your thoughts. Start by writing down a painful thought as it arises, then note the emotions it triggers and the behaviors it prompts. Next, examine the evidence for and against this thought, considering alternative, more balanced interpretations. This reflective process allows you to confront and reframe negative thoughts, reducing their hold over your emotions and actions. Another effective strategy is practicing gratitude. By regularly reflecting on aspects of your life that you appreciate, you shift your focus away from pain, fostering a more positive outlook. This practice enhances your emotional well-being and creates a buffer against the stress and negativity that can exacerbate physical symptoms.

CBT plays a vital role in chronic pain management, offering a holistic approach that complements physical treatments. It emphasizes the mind-body connection, recognizing that how you think and feel can influence your physical well-being. Numerous case studies highlight the success of CBT in managing chronic pain. Take the example of Mark, a middle-aged professional who struggled with debilitating neck pain for years. Through CBT, he learned to identify the catastrophic thoughts that amplified his pain and replaced them with more balanced, constructive ones. As a result, Mark experienced a significant reduction in pain intensity and an improvement in his quality of life. His story illustrates the transformative power of CBT, demonstrating how changing your mindset can lead to tangible improvements in physical health.

For those seeking personalized guidance, collaborating with a therapist skilled in CBT can be incredibly beneficial. A professional can tailor strategies to your unique needs, offering insights and techniques that you might not discover on your own. They can guide you through exercises, provide feedback, and help you navigate challenges, ensuring that you make the most of your CBT practice. Engaging with a therapist also provides a supportive environment to explore and address underlying issues that may contribute to your pain, fostering a comprehensive approach to healing. While CBT offers valuable techniques for self-management, the support of a professional can enhance your journey, providing the encouragement and expertise needed to effect lasting change.

6.3 VISUALIZATION TECHNIQUES FOR ENHANCED RECOVERY

Visualization harnesses the power of mental imagery, offering a profound way to enhance recovery and manage pain. By engaging your mind in the process of healing, visualization taps into the body's natural capacity to respond to positive mental cues. Imagine visualizing your neck as free of pain, each muscle relaxed and each movement fluid. This mental imagery acts as a catalyst for physical change, encouraging your muscles to release tension and promoting an overall sense of well-being. The technique is not just about imagining the absence of pain; it's about creating a clear mental picture of what healing looks like, reinforcing the body's natural repair processes. Visualization becomes a tool for motivation, empowering you to see beyond the immediate discomfort and envision a future where pain no longer dictates your actions.

To effectively integrate visualization into your daily practice, consider specific exercises that support neck health. Start with imagining a pain-free neck as a source of motivation. Close your eyes and visualize your neck moving effortlessly, free from stiffness or discomfort. Picture each vertebra aligned perfectly, each muscle supporting gentle, fluid motion. This imagery can serve as a powerful motivator, especially during challenging moments when pain seems overwhelming. By focusing on this ideal state, you reinforce the belief that recovery is achievable, fostering resilience and determination. Another technique involves visualizing muscle relaxation during stressful moments. When you feel tension creeping in, close your eyes and imagine your neck muscles softening and lengthening. Picture the tension melting away with each breath, replaced by a sense of calm and ease. This practice not only alleviates immediate discomfort but also trains your body to respond to stress with relaxation rather than contraction.

Beyond pain relief, visualization offers benefits that extend into various aspects of life, enhancing overall well-being and motivation. Through regular practice, you can cultivate enhanced focus and concentration. Visualization demands a level of mental discipline and clarity that translates into other areas of life. As you hone this skill, you may notice improved attention and productivity in daily tasks. The practice also fosters a positive mindset, helping you maintain motivation even when progress seems slow. By regularly envisioning your goals and the steps to achieve them, you reinforce a sense of purpose and drive. This mental rehearsal builds confidence, making challenges feel more manageable and goals more attainable.

Incorporating visualization into your daily routine can be both simple and rewarding. Consider starting your day with a morning visualization session, setting a positive tone for the hours ahead. Find a quiet space where you won't be disturbed, and close your eyes. Take a few deep breaths to center yourself, then begin visualizing your neck moving with ease and without pain. Allow this imagery to fill your mind, focusing on the sensations of freedom and comfort. This practice not only primes your mind for the day but also reinforces your commitment to recovery. Visualization can be woven into other moments as well—during a commute, while waiting in line, or before falling asleep. Each session reinforces your body's healing capacity, creating a consistent and powerful support system for neck health.

Visualization is more than a mental exercise; it's a bridge between your mind and body, facilitating communication that supports healing and growth. By engaging in this practice, you empower yourself to play an active role in your recovery, using the power of your mind to influence your physical state. Whether you're dealing with chronic neck pain or seeking to enhance overall wellness, visualization offers a pathway to resilience, clarity, and healing.

6.4 JOURNALING FOR PAIN MANAGEMENT: TRACKING PROGRESS AND TRIGGERS

Journaling emerges as a powerful therapeutic tool, offering a unique way to track pain patterns and emotional triggers. When you write about your experiences, you begin to uncover connections between your daily activities, emotional states, and the intensity of your neck pain. This process of self-reflection allows you to identify specific stressors that might be contributing to your discomfort. For instance, you may discover that certain work-related tasks consistently lead to tension in your neck, or that emotional stress from personal relationships exacerbates your pain. By documenting these insights, you gain clarity, enabling you to make informed decisions about how to better manage your pain. Journaling becomes a mirror, reflecting your inner thoughts and external circumstances, providing a comprehensive view of your pain journey.

To maximize the benefits of journaling, employing effective techniques can guide you in capturing meaningful insights. Daily pain and mood logs serve as a foundational tool, offering a structured way to record your experiences. Each day, take a few moments to note the level of pain you experience, along with any significant events or emotions. Over time, these logs reveal patterns, helping you pinpoint triggers and track progress. Reflective questions can further deepen your understanding. Consider questions like, "What emotions am I feeling today, and how do they relate to my neck pain?" or "What activities or thoughts seem to alleviate or worsen my pain?" These prompts encourage self-discovery, allowing you to delve beneath the surface and uncover hidden connections.

The benefits of journaling extend far beyond simply tracking pain. This practice fosters increased self-awareness, encouraging you to engage with your thoughts and emotions on a deeper level. As you write, you process your feelings, facilitating emotional release and reducing the mental burden associated with chronic pain. Journaling also supports mental health, acting as a safe space where you can express your frustrations, fears, and victories. This outlet for emotional processing helps alleviate stress, which can in turn reduce physical tension in your neck. By regularly engaging in this practice, you cultivate a greater sense of control over your well-being, empowering you to take proactive steps toward healing.

Consistency is key to reaping the full benefits of journaling. Set aside dedicated time each day or week to engage in this reflective practice. Whether it's in the morning with a cup of coffee or before bed as you wind down, find a time that suits your routine and encourages regular reflection. Creating a comforting journaling space can enhance the experience. Choose a quiet corner of your home, perhaps adorned with calming elements like a soft chair or ambient lighting. This space becomes a sanctuary, inviting you to explore your thoughts without distraction. Keep your journal and writing tools easily accessible, ensuring that you can capture insights whenever they arise.

As you continue to journal, you'll find that this practice supports your neck health and enriches your overall well-being. The act of writing bridges the gap between your mind and body, fostering a holistic approach to pain management. By engaging in regular reflection, you gain a clearer understanding of your experiences, empowering you to navigate the challenges of neck pain with greater resilience. Journaling offers a sense of continuity, a thread that weaves through your daily life, connecting each moment with the next. Through this practice, you create a narrative of healing and growth, one that unfolds with each entry you write, guiding you toward a more balanced and fulfilling life.

6.5 BUILDING A SUPPORT SYSTEM: ENCOURAGING COMMUNITY AND CONNECTION

Navigating the complexities of neck pain often feels like an isolating experience, yet it's one shared by many. Establishing a robust support system can profoundly impact both your mental health and your journey to managing pain. When you connect with others who understand your challenges, it transforms the experience from one of solitude to shared resilience. Sharing your experiences with others can reduce feelings of isolation, creating a sense of belonging and mutual understanding. Knowing that someone else has walked a similar path can be comforting, offering emotional relief and practical insights.

Joining support groups or online forums dedicated to neck pain management can be immensely beneficial. These communities offer a space to exchange advice, share personal stories, and offer encouragement. Through platforms like these, you can gain access to a wealth of collective wisdom, learning from others' successes and setbacks. Participating in discussions can also provide motivation, showing you that progress is possible. Additionally, these groups often include members who have tried various treatments, providing firsthand reviews and recommendations that can guide your decisions.

Open communication with friends and family is equally important. Sometimes, those closest to you may not fully grasp the extent of your pain, but by sharing your experiences and challenges, you foster empathy and support. Honest conversations can lead to practical assistance, such as help with daily tasks or emotional support during difficult times. Encouraging open dialogue about your struggles strengthens your relationships and creates an environment where you feel safe and understood. This emotional backing can significantly enhance your ability to cope with pain, reducing stress and improving your overall well-being.

Professional support should not be overlooked in building a comprehensive support network. Consulting with healthcare professionals, such as mental health counselors, can provide valuable insights into managing both the emotional and physical aspects of pain. Counselors offer strategies to cope with stress and anxiety, which can otherwise exacerbate neck pain. Engaging with physical therapists can provide holistic care, addressing the physical components of your condition. These professionals can tailor treatment plans to your specific needs, offering exercises and techniques that promote healing and prevent further injury. Their expertise and guidance can be instrumental in achieving lasting relief.

Community engagement offers another dimension to building a support network, fostering connection and purpose beyond individual struggles. Participating in community activities, such as volunteering, can provide a sense of fulfillment and belonging. These activities distract from the focus on pain and create opportunities to meet new people and form meaningful connections. Volunteering, in particular, allows you to contribute to causes you care about, enhancing your sense of purpose and boosting your mood. The benefits of community involvement extend beyond the immediate, often leading to lasting friendships and a strengthened support network.

As you explore these avenues for building support, remember that the journey is personal, and each step you take is significant. By reaching out and connecting with others, you create a foundation of strength and resilience that supports your health and well-being. This chapter illuminates the ways in which mental wellness and community can intersect, offering a holistic approach to managing neck pain. As we transition to the next chapter, we will delve into maintaining motivation and tracking progress, further equipping you with the tools to navigate your path to recovery.

7

MAINTAINING MOTIVATION AND TRACKING PROGRESS

Picture yourself standing at the edge of a vast, open field, the morning sun casting a warm glow as you prepare for a new day. In this field, you can plant the seeds of your recovery journey. These seeds represent your goals—each one a step towards overcoming neck pain. Setting realistic goals is like mapping a path through this field, guiding you towards the relief and vitality you seek. Goals provide structure and motivation, transforming aspirations into tangible achievements. Without them, the path can seem nebulous and overwhelming. By clearly defining what you want to achieve, you illuminate the way forward, making each step purposeful and focused.

The distinction between short-term and long-term goals is essential. Short-term goals act as stepping stones, offering immediate targets that keep your motivation high. These might include mastering a particular stretch or maintaining a consistent exercise routine for a month. Long-term goals, on the other hand, are the overarching achievements you strive towards, such as living a pain-free life or returning to a beloved sport. Aligning these goals with your personal values and lifestyle ensures they resonate deeply with you, fostering a genuine commitment to your recovery. For instance, if you value health and well-being, your goals might focus on integrating holistic practices that support both physical and mental health.

Creating a personalized recovery plan involves setting goals that are Specific, Measurable, Achievable, Relevant, and Time-bound (SMART). This framework provides clarity and direction, ensuring your goals are both challenging and attainable. Begin by identifying what you specifically want to achieve, whether it's reducing pain intensity or improving neck flexibility. Make these goals measurable by defining the criteria for success, such as performing a set of exercises without discomfort. Ensure your goals are achievable, taking into account your current abilities and resources. Relevance is key; your goals should align with your broader life objectives and values. Finally, set a clear timeframe for achieving each goal, providing a sense of urgency and focus.

As you embark on your recovery, it's important to prioritize goals based on your current needs and abilities. Consider what is most urgent or impactful for your well-being, and let that guide your focus. Flexibility in goal setting is crucial, as progress is rarely linear. Life circumstances change, and setbacks occur—what matters is your ability to adapt. Adjust your goals as needed, whether by extending timelines, modifying targets, or redefining success. This adaptability ensures that your recovery plan remains relevant and realistic, keeping you engaged and motivated.

Visualization techniques can reinforce your commitment to goal achievement. Mental imagery allows you to picture successful outcomes, harnessing the power of your mind to enhance motivation. Visualize yourself completing exercises with ease, experiencing the freedom of movement without pain. This imagery boosts confidence and conditions your mind for success. By regularly engaging in visualization, you create a mental blueprint for your achievements, making the abstract tangible and attainable.

Interactive Element: Goal-Setting Worksheet

Reflect on your personal goals and use the following questions to develop a SMART recovery plan:

1. **Specific**: What exactly do you want to achieve in your neck pain recovery?
2. **Measurable**: How will you know when you've reached your goal? What indicators will show progress?
3. **Achievable**: Is this goal realistic given your current resources and abilities?
4. **Relevant**: How does this goal align with your broader life values and objectives?
5. **Time-bound**: By when do you want to achieve this goal?

Take a moment to write down your answers and create a clear, actionable plan that guides your recovery journey.

By thoughtfully setting and pursuing goals, you lay a strong foundation for a successful recovery. Embrace the journey with a sense of purpose, knowing that each step brings you closer to the vibrant, pain-free life you envision.

7.1 MONITORING YOUR PROGRESS: TOOLS AND TECHNIQUES FOR TRACKING IMPROVEMENT

Imagine navigating a long road without markers or signs, uncertain about your distance or direction. Progress tracking serves as those essential markers, illuminating where you've been and where you're headed. It reinforces positive habits by providing tangible evidence of your achievements, an often-overlooked aspect of motivation. When you see your efforts translated into measurable progress, it fuels your determination to persist. This visibility makes each small victory a stepping stone, reinforcing the behaviors necessary for sustained recovery. The sense of accomplishment derived from seeing your progress propels you forward, transforming abstract goals into concrete achievements.

A variety of tools and techniques are at your disposal to monitor both physical and mental improvements. Journals and diaries offer a personal space for reflection, allowing you to document daily experiences, challenges, and successes. This narrative not only tracks your physical progress but also captures emotional and psychological growth. Digital apps, on the other hand, provide a structured way to track exercise routines and pain levels. Apps like Fitbit or EXi, which integrate with devices to monitor activity and health metrics, can provide detailed insights into your progress. These digital tools offer convenience and precision, making it easier to identify patterns and areas for improvement. Progress charts offer a visual representation of your journey, making it easy to spot trends and track milestones. Watching a chart's line climb upward can be incredibly motivating, showing you that your efforts are yielding results.

Feedback plays a crucial role in effective progress tracking. Regular self-assessment check-ins help you evaluate what's working and what needs adjustment. These check-ins can be as simple as asking yourself questions about your pain levels or reflecting on how you feel after certain exercises. By periodically reviewing your progress, you gain valuable insights into your recovery, allowing for adjustments that enhance effectiveness. Such feedback loops ensure that your efforts remain aligned with your goals, promoting efficiency and focus. This practice of self-assessment fosters a proactive attitude, encouraging you to take ownership of your recovery.

Consistent evaluations, such as monthly progress summaries, provide a broader view of your journey. By taking time each month to review your achievements and challenges, you maintain focus and motivation. These evaluations serve as a reality check, reminding you of how far you've come and what lies ahead. They offer an opportunity to celebrate successes, however small, and to recalibrate your approach if necessary. Regular reviews ensure that your recovery plan remains dynamic and responsive to your evolving needs. They help you stay on track, preventing stagnation and complacency.

Interactive Element: Progress Tracking Template

Consider using the following template to structure your tracking efforts:

1. **Daily Reflections**: Note down any significant changes in pain levels, mood, or energy.
2. **Weekly Highlights**: Summarize key achievements or setbacks from the week.
3. **Monthly Summary**: Review overall progress, focusing on patterns and trends.
4. **Feedback Note**: Identify areas for improvement and adjust your plan accordingly.

By consistently monitoring your progress, you build a detailed map of your recovery. This map not only guides your actions but also inspires confidence in your ability to achieve lasting relief.

7.2 STAYING MOTIVATED: TIPS FOR OVERCOMING PLATEAUS AND SETBACKS

In the pursuit of neck pain relief, maintaining motivation can feel like an uphill battle. The initial enthusiasm often wanes as the challenges of sustaining progress become apparent. One common obstacle is the plateau, where improvements stagnate and the frustration of perceived inertia takes root. It's the emotional weight of working hard yet feeling stuck that can dampen spirits. You might find yourself questioning the efficacy of your efforts, wondering why the pain persists despite your dedication. This is a natural part of recovery, yet it doesn't make it any less discouraging. Recognizing this struggle is the first step in overcoming it, as acknowledging the difficulty allows you to address it directly.

When faced with a plateau, introducing variety into your exercise routine can breathe new life into your regimen. Your body adapts to repetitive actions, which can diminish their impact over time. By diversifying your exercises, you challenge different muscle groups, preventing adaptation and promoting growth. Consider incorporating new activities that align with your interests or exploring variations of existing exercises. This reinvigorates your routine and keeps your mind engaged, reducing the monotony that can lead to disengagement. Alongside this, setting new, smaller goals can rekindle motivation by providing immediate targets to strive for. These mini-goals act as markers of progress, offering a sense of achievement and momentum. Whether it's increasing the duration of a stretch or mastering a new technique, these incremental victories build confidence and enthusiasm.

The power of mindset in overcoming setbacks cannot be overstated. Cultivating positive thinking and resilience transforms challenges into opportunities for growth. Instead of viewing setbacks as failures, consider them as learning experiences. This reframing shifts your perspective, encouraging a proactive approach to problem-solving. When a particular exercise exacerbates pain, it becomes a chance to reassess your technique or explore alternative methods. Embracing setbacks with curiosity rather than frustration fosters a resilient mindset, which is essential for long-term recovery. This mental shift enhances your ability to adapt, ensuring that obstacles become stepping stones rather than roadblocks.

During difficult times, seeking support from others can provide the encouragement and fresh perspectives needed to push through. Connecting with a mentor or coach offers guidance and reassurance. These individuals bring experience and insight, helping you navigate the complexities of recovery. Their external perspective can identify areas for improvement that you might overlook, offering tailored advice to enhance your approach. Additionally, reaching out to peers who share similar experiences fosters a sense of community and understanding. Shared stories of triumphs and challenges create a support network that bolsters your motivation, reminding you that you're not alone in this journey.

In moments of doubt, remember that setbacks are a natural part of any meaningful endeavor. They test your resolve, but they also provide the impetus for growth and improvement. The path to recovery is rarely linear, and it's through these challenges that resilience is forged. By embracing variety, setting achievable goals, cultivating a positive mindset, and seeking support, you equip yourself with the tools to not only overcome plateaus but to thrive beyond them. Let the spirit of perseverance guide you, turning obstacles into opportunities and transforming the process of recovery into one of empowerment and renewal.

7.3 CELEBRATING MILESTONES: RECOGNIZING ACHIEVEMENTS ON YOUR JOURNEY

Imagine the satisfaction of reaching the summit of a mountain after a long and arduous climb. Celebrating milestones in your recovery journey serves a similar purpose. It acknowledges your achievements and reinforces the progress you've made. Recognizing these moments boosts your confidence, reminding you that every effort counts. The act of celebration is more than just a pat on the back; it's a powerful psychological tool that enhances motivation and commitment. When you celebrate, you affirm the value of your hard work, which can fuel your drive to keep pushing forward. This sense of accomplishment creates a positive feedback loop, encouraging you to maintain your focus and dedication.

There are many creative ways to celebrate your personal achievements in recovery. Perhaps you could reward yourself with a small treat or experience that brings you joy. It can be as simple as a favorite meal, a new book, or a relaxing day at the spa. These rewards act as tangible reminders of your success, creating a link between effort and enjoyment. Sharing your victories with friends or support groups can also amplify the joy of your accomplishments. Whether it's a heartfelt post on social media or a call to a close friend, sharing your progress allows others to join in your celebration and provide encouragement. This sense of community support can strengthen your resolve and inspire those around you.

Reflection is a key component of celebrating milestones. Taking time to reflect on how far you've come and the obstacles you've overcome helps solidify your achievements in your mind. Writing a reflective journal entry about your accomplishments allows you to articulate your progress and the lessons learned along the way. This reflection deepens your understanding of your journey and provides a record of your transformation. It serves as a personal testament to your resilience and determination, one you can revisit whenever you need a reminder of your capabilities. Through reflection, you gain insight into the strategies that worked well and the challenges you navigated, empowering you to apply these insights to future goals.

Celebrating milestones has a profound impact on long-term motivation. Each celebration strengthens your commitment to ongoing goals by creating positive associations with achievement. The anticipation of future celebrations can serve as a motivational beacon, guiding you through difficult times. When you associate success with positive emotions and rewards, you reinforce the behaviors that lead to those outcomes. This reinforcement encourages consistency and perseverance, which are crucial for sustained progress. As you celebrate each milestone, you build a foundation of confidence and optimism, enabling you to approach new challenges with a positive mindset.

In the context of recovery, celebration is not merely an endpoint but an integral part of the process. It transforms the journey into a series of meaningful achievements, each one a stepping stone towards your ultimate goal. By celebrating your milestones, you acknowledge the effort and dedication that brought you to this point, while also paving the way for future successes. Embrace these moments of celebration as opportunities to honor your progress and reaffirm your commitment to your recovery journey.

7.4 CREATING A ROUTINE: INTEGRATING EXERCISES INTO DAILY LIFE

Imagine the rhythm of your daily life as a dance, where each step is deliberate and contributes to the overall harmony. Just as a dancer relies on muscle memory to glide effortlessly across the stage, incorporating a consistent exercise routine into your daily life builds a similar foundation for recovery. Regular practice establishes a rhythm that your body comes to expect, enhancing your recovery and minimizing setbacks. When you engage in exercises consistently, you reinforce neural pathways and improve muscle memory, making each movement more natural and less prone to error. This familiarity reduces the mental and physical effort required, allowing you to focus on refining your technique and achieving optimal results.

The key to integrating exercises into your daily routine lies in making them as natural as possible. Start by scheduling specific times for your exercises, treating them as non-negotiable appointments with yourself. This commitment ensures that your exercises become a habitual part of your day rather than an afterthought. Consider the moments in your daily routine where exercises can seamlessly fit, such as stretching while watching TV or doing neck exercises during a work break. By aligning exercises with existing activities, you create a synergy that minimizes disruption and maximizes efficiency. These moments of multitasking enhance your physical well-being and provide a mental break, allowing you to return to your tasks with renewed focus and energy.

Habit formation plays a critical role in simplifying adherence to exercise routines. Habits are powerful because they don't require conscious effort or motivation; they become automatic behaviors that you perform without thinking. To cultivate these habits, use triggers to prompt your exercise sessions. A trigger could be as simple as setting an alarm or associating your exercises with a specific event, like brushing your teeth or finishing a meal. Over time, these triggers act as cues, signaling your body to prepare for exercise and reinforcing the habit loop. As the habit strengthens, it becomes easier to maintain consistency, even on days when motivation wanes.

Gradual integration is crucial for building a sustainable routine. Starting small allows you to ease into the habit without feeling overwhelmed. Begin with a simple 5-minute daily routine, focusing on basic exercises that target key areas like the neck and shoulders. This short duration makes it easy to commit, ensuring that you can fit the exercises into even the busiest of days. As your confidence and comfort grow, gradually increase the complexity and duration of your routines. This incremental approach prevents burnout and allows your body to adapt, reducing the risk of injury and fostering long-term adherence. By taking small, manageable steps, you create a solid foundation for a lifelong commitment to health and wellness.

In this dance of routine, the steps you take are not just about physical movement but about creating a rhythm that aligns with your life. Each repetition, each stretch, and each moment of mindfulness contributes to the choreography of your recovery. Embrace the process, knowing that every step forward is a step towards a healthier, more resilient you.

7.5 THE ROLE OF ACCOUNTABILITY: FINDING A PARTNER OR GROUP FOR SUPPORT

Imagine being on a long hike, the path winding through dense forests and over challenging terrains. Having a companion by your side makes the journey more enjoyable and provides that extra push when you feel like giving up. In the realm of recovery, accountability serves a similar purpose. It acts as a motivational tool that enhances your commitment to your goals, especially when the going gets tough. An accountability partner or group brings shared goals into the picture, creating a collective energy that propels everyone forward. This shared motivation can significantly increase your sense of responsibility and drive, making the process of recovery less daunting and more collaborative.

Finding the right accountability partner or group involves identifying individuals who share your commitment to recovery and well-being. Start by exploring local exercise or wellness groups, where like-minded individuals gather with similar goals. These groups offer a sense of community and support, making it easier to connect with others who understand your challenges. Alternatively, consider partnering with a friend or family member who shares your enthusiasm for health and fitness. Their presence can offer encouragement, creating a supportive environment where you feel understood and motivated. The key is to find someone whose goals align with yours, ensuring that your partnership reinforces your commitment to recovery.

The benefits of shared experiences in recovery are immense. When you share your journey with others, you open the door to encouragement and fresh insights. This exchange of ideas and experiences can be incredibly empowering, as you learn from others' successes and challenges. Sharing challenges with a group fosters a sense of camaraderie, where you realize that you're not alone in your struggles. This collective support can alleviate feelings of isolation, providing the reassurance that others are walking a similar path. Additionally, discussing solutions with others can spark new strategies for overcoming obstacles, enhancing your approach to recovery.

To ensure that your accountability relationships are supportive and beneficial, consider implementing strategies that foster effective collaboration. Set regular check-ins with your partner or group to discuss progress, share achievements, and address any setbacks. These check-ins create a structured framework for accountability, encouraging consistent engagement and reflection.

Progress updates can be as simple as a weekly call or message, where you celebrate wins and discuss areas for improvement. By maintaining open communication, you cultivate a supportive environment that promotes honesty and growth. This transparency builds trust, strengthening the bond between you and your accountability partner.

Incorporating accountability into your recovery plan transforms the process from a solitary endeavor into a shared experience. It leverages the power of community to enhance motivation, making the path to recovery more engaging and rewarding. With a partner or group by your side, you gain access to a wealth of perspectives and support, enriching your journey with empathy and encouragement. As you move forward, remember that accountability is not just about meeting goals; it's about fostering connections that inspire and uplift. These connections become a source of strength, empowering you to face challenges with confidence and resilience.

In this chapter, we explored various strategies for maintaining motivation and tracking progress, emphasizing the importance of accountability in enhancing commitment. As you integrate these practices into your recovery, you'll find that each step brings you closer to your goals. Next, we will delve into the specifics of implementing lifestyle changes that support neck health, building on the foundation of motivation and accountability established here.

8

SUCCESS STORIES AND PROFESSIONAL INSIGHTS

Imagine waking up one morning, the familiar weight of neck pain absent, and in its place, a newfound sense of freedom. This is not just a dream but a reality for many who have embraced the strategies outlined in this book. In this chapter, you will discover compelling stories of individuals from diverse backgrounds who have reclaimed their lives from the grip of neck pain. Their journeys reflect not only the challenges they faced but also the triumphs that come with perseverance and the right approach. These narratives are more than just anecdotes; they are testaments to the power of targeted exercises, lifestyle modifications, and mental wellness techniques.

Consider the story of James, a dedicated professional whose life revolved around his demanding office job. Hours hunched over a computer had taken a toll, leaving him with persistent neck pain that shadowed him day and night. Skeptical at first, James began implementing ergonomic adjustments to his workstation. By elevating his monitor and investing in an adjustable chair, he transformed his desk into a haven for neck health. Gradually, the pain that had once seemed insurmountable began to recede. "It was like peeling away layers of discomfort," James reflects. "Each adjustment made a difference, and over time, the relief was profound." His story is a beacon of hope for those trapped in similar cycles of pain, proving that small changes can lead to significant improvements.

In the realm of athletics, where peak performance is paramount, neck pain can be a formidable adversary. Take Maria, a competitive swimmer whose rigorous training regimen left her with chronic pain that threatened her career. Through targeted exercises focusing on neck and shoulder stability, Maria found her way back to the pool with renewed vigor. By incorporating resistance band workouts and dynamic stretching into her routine, she alleviated her pain and enhanced her overall performance. "The exercises were my lifeline," Maria shares. "They didn't just relieve the pain; they made me stronger." Her journey underscores the importance of tailored exercise programs in overcoming physical limitations, especially for athletes committed to their craft.

For many, the demands of parenting are relentless, and the added burden of neck pain can seem overwhelming. Sarah, a mother of three, faced this challenge head-on. Her days were a whirlwind of activity, leaving little time for self-care. Yet, through mindfulness and stress reduction practices, Sarah discovered a transformative path to relief. By dedicating just a few minutes each day to deep breathing and meditation, she found a sanctuary amidst the chaos. "Mindfulness was my escape," Sarah explains. "It allowed me to step back and breathe, easing the tension that had built up." Her story is a testament to the power of mental wellness techniques in managing physical pain, offering a roadmap for others seeking balance in their busy lives.

These stories represent just a fraction of the diverse experiences shared by individuals who have embraced change and found relief from neck pain. They come from various age groups and lifestyles, each with unique obstacles and triumphs. Some faced initial skepticism, questioning the efficacy of new approaches. Yet, as they persisted, the gradual improvements became undeniable. Their personal reflections reveal the depth of their struggles and the profound impact that overcoming neck pain has had on their lives. "Living without pain has given me back my life," one individual notes. "I feel empowered, capable of taking on challenges I once thought impossible." Through their words, we gain insight into the transformative power of the strategies detailed in this book.

Reflective Exercise

Consider your own journey with neck pain. What small changes can you make today to start on the path to relief? Reflect on the stories shared in this chapter and identify one strategy that resonates with you. Write down your thoughts and commit to trying it for a week. Reassess your progress and adjust as needed, knowing that each step forward is a victory in itself.

These narratives are woven with authenticity and resilience, illustrating the profound difference that the right strategies can make. They inspire action and reinforce the message that relief is within reach, no matter the hurdles.

8.1 EXPERT INTERVIEWS: INSIGHTS FROM CHIROPRACTORS AND PHYSICAL THERAPISTS

Within the realm of neck pain management, chiropractors and physical therapists emerge as pivotal voices, offering insights that blend clinical expertise with practical wisdom. In conversations with seasoned chiropractors and physical therapists, the consensus is clear: neck spinal posture and exercise stands as a cornerstone in the fight against neck pain. They emphasize that targeted adjustments and exercises alleviate discomfort and fortify the neck's supportive structures. They highlighted the importance of consistent practice, particularly with movements that enhance flexibility and strength. "Think of your neck as a complex machine," and "Regular maintenance through optimal alignment and exercise keeps it functioning smoothly." This advice resonates especially with those who have experienced the crippling effects of inactivity, underscoring the transformative power of movement.

Equally compelling are the perspectives shared by spine doctors who advocate for lifestyle changes as integral to recovery. They point to the interconnectedness of physical health and daily habits, noting how poor posture and unhealthy routines can exacerbate neck pain. One doctor shared a compelling observation: "Patients often overlook the impact of their daily environment on their neck health." He recommended simple adjustments, such as ensuring ergonomic setups at workstations and practicing good posture throughout daily activities. By addressing these foundational elements, patients often find relief that medication alone cannot provide. These insights serve as a reminder that recovery is not just about addressing symptoms but also about creating an environment that supports long-term health.

Professionals also stress the role of mental wellness in comprehensive care. They assert that a holistic approach, which includes mental health practices, can significantly enhance physical recovery. Mindfulness and stress reduction techniques, like meditation and deep breathing, are often recommended alongside physical therapies. According to one expert, "When the mind is calm, the body follows suit." This approach aligns with the book's philosophy, emphasizing the need to address both mental and physical aspects of health to achieve sustainable relief from neck pain. The integration of these practices helps patients build resilience against stress-induced muscle tension, a common trigger for neck discomfort.

As discussions with these experts unfold, a pattern emerges: combining traditional therapy with holistic practices yields the most effective results. This integration is not merely a trend, but a necessary evolution in treating neck pain. Experts advocate for methods that marry the best of both worlds, allowing for personalized care that adapts to individual needs. One physiotherapist explained, "Incorporating holistic elements into traditional treatment plans empowers patients, giving them the tools to manage their health proactively." This synergy of approaches resonates with those seeking a well-rounded path to recovery, providing a framework that supports both immediate relief and long-term wellness.

Drawing from these expert insights, several practical tips can be implemented immediately. Key exercises such as chin tucks, shoulder rolls, and gentle neck stretches are highly recommended. These movements aid in maintaining flexibility and reducing tension. The therapists stress the importance of integrating these exercises into daily routines, even suggesting setting reminders to perform them regularly. Additionally, they emphasize the value of mindfulness techniques, encouraging readers to carve out moments for relaxation and reflection. These small but impactful changes, endorsed by leading professionals, offer a proactive path toward relief and a healthier neck.

8.2 THE SCIENCE BEHIND THE SOLUTIONS: EVIDENCE SUPPORTING OUR APPROACH

Understanding the science behind neck pain management provides a solid foundation for the strategies within this book. Extensive research supports the efficacy of ergonomic interventions in reducing neck pain. Studies consistently demonstrate that proper ergonomic setups, such as adjustable chairs and correctly positioned monitors, significantly decrease the strain on cervical structures. By aligning the body in a natural posture, these adjustments reduce muscle fatigue and prevent the onset of pain. This is not merely anecdotal; data from multiple studies reveal a marked improvement in pain levels among those who adopted ergonomic changes in their work environments. For instance, one study found that individuals who utilized ergonomic workstations reported a 50% reduction in neck pain over six months. Such statistics underscore the transformative potential of ergonomic interventions in daily life.

Beyond physical adjustments, the role of mindfulness in pain reduction has garnered substantial scientific backing. Mindfulness practices, which focus on present-moment awareness and stress reduction, have been shown to decrease the perception of pain. Research indicates that regular mindfulness meditation can alter the way the brain processes pain signals, reducing their intensity and frequency. In one study, participants who engaged in mindfulness techniques reported a 30% reduction in pain intensity. This effect is attributed to mindfulness's ability to modulate stress responses, thereby easing tension in the neck and shoulders. These findings highlight the importance of integrating mental wellness practices into physical health routines, creating a holistic approach to neck pain management.

The mechanisms through which exercises alleviate neck pain are rooted in basic anatomical principles. Targeted exercises strengthen the muscles that support the cervical spine, enhancing stability and range of motion. By fortifying these muscles, exercises help prevent the micro-injuries that often lead to chronic pain. Moreover, strengthening exercises promote better posture, reducing undue pressure on the neck. This dual action of support and correction is why exercises are a cornerstone of effective neck pain management. A study published in a leading medical journal showed that participants who engaged in regular neck-strengthening exercises experienced a 40% improvement in pain scores, emphasizing the tangible benefits of physical activity.

Stress reduction plays a critical role in alleviating neck pain, as chronic stress activates physiological processes that exacerbate discomfort. When stress levels rise, the body releases cortisol, a hormone that increases muscle tension and inflammation. Prolonged stress can lead to persistent neck pain, as tense muscles become more susceptible to injury. By employing stress reduction techniques, such as deep breathing and progressive muscle relaxation, individuals can lower cortisol levels, thereby reducing muscle tightness and pain. This physiological shift illustrates the intricate connection between mental and physical health, reinforcing the need for comprehensive strategies that address both aspects.

To reinforce the credibility of these approaches, it is essential to reference peer-reviewed studies and articles. Scholarly research has consistently supported the strategies outlined in this book, providing a robust evidence base for their efficacy. For example, a comprehensive review of ergonomic interventions published in the Journal of Occupational Health found significant reductions in musculoskeletal pain among office workers who implemented ergonomic changes.

Similarly, a study in the Journal of Pain Research affirmed the benefits of mindfulness, showing that participants experienced a notable decrease in pain perception and an increase in pain tolerance. These sources lend authority to the recommendations provided, offering reassurance that they are grounded in scientific rigor.

The effectiveness of these strategies is not just theoretical but proven through empirical evidence. By integrating ergonomic adjustments, mindfulness practices, and targeted exercises, individuals can achieve significant relief from neck pain. The data speaks volumes, highlighting the potential for meaningful change through informed action. This scientific foundation validates the approaches within this book and empowers you with the knowledge to take charge of your neck health.

8.3 COMMON PITFALLS AND HOW TO AVOID THEM: LEARNING FROM OTHERS' MISTAKES

Navigating the intricacies of neck pain management can often seem like walking a tightrope. It requires balance and mindfulness to avoid the common pitfalls that many encounter. One significant misstep is ignoring posture until the situation becomes severe. Many individuals continue their daily routines, unaware of the strain they place on their neck, until the pain is too intense to ignore. This negligence often stems from the misconception that only drastic measures can alleviate discomfort. However, by the time the pain becomes unbearable, the damage may have already set in, making recovery more challenging. This highlights the importance of early intervention and consistent attention to posture.

Another frequent error is relying heavily on medication to mask symptoms without addressing root causes. While painkillers offer temporary relief, they don't solve the underlying issues. Over time, this approach can lead to an overreliance on medication, which may be accompanied by side effects and diminishing effectiveness. Instead, incorporating strategies like targeted exercises and ergonomic adjustments can tackle the core of the problem. These methods promote healing by strengthening and supporting the neck's structures. By taking proactive measures, you can reduce dependency on medication and improve overall neck health.

Establishing a consistent routine is a powerful antidote to these pitfalls. Regularly practicing neck exercises and maintaining ergonomic habits can prevent the onset of pain. Consistency also reinforces positive behaviors, creating a protective barrier against future discomfort. Alongside this, seeking professional guidance when needed can provide clarity and direction. Healthcare professionals offer tailored advice, ensuring that your approach to neck pain management is both effective and personalized. Their expertise can help you navigate the nuances of your condition, offering insights that empower you to make informed decisions.

Consider the story of Alex, who found himself at a plateau after months of self-directed care. Initially, Alex experienced significant relief by incorporating exercises into his daily routine. However, progress stalled, and frustration set in. Recognizing the need for a fresh perspective, he consulted a physical chiropractor, who identified areas needing adjustment. With slight modifications to his exercise regimen and posture, Alex broke through the plateau and continued to improve. His experience underscores the importance of adaptability and seeking external input when faced with stagnation.

Persistence is an invaluable trait in the quest for neck pain relief. Challenges and setbacks are inevitable, yet they are not insurmountable. Embracing patience and adaptability can guide you through these hurdles. The path to recovery is rarely linear, but each obstacle presents an opportunity to learn and grow. By maintaining a steadfast commitment to your health, you can cultivate resilience and determination. These qualities will serve as allies, propelling you toward long-term success and a life less burdened by pain.

It's important to remember that the management of neck pain is both a personal and evolving process. It requires continuous engagement and a willingness to adjust strategies as needed. By learning from the mistakes of others and applying these lessons, you can avoid common pitfalls and set yourself on a path to sustained improvement.

8.4 THE FUTURE OF NECK PAIN MANAGEMENT: EMERGING TRENDS AND TECHNOLOGIES

In the fast-paced world of healthcare, the management of neck pain is evolving rapidly, driven by innovative treatments and cutting-edge technologies. One prominent development is the rise of wearable technology, which is transforming the way individuals monitor and manage their posture. Devices like smart posture correctors provide real-time feedback on body alignment, gently vibrating to remind users to maintain proper posture. This immediate feedback loop empowers users to make adjustments before discomfort sets in, fostering healthy habits that can significantly reduce the incidence of neck pain. By integrating these wearables into daily routines, individuals are equipped with the tools to proactively manage their neck health, embracing a future where prevention is as vital as treatment.

The landscape of healthcare is also being reshaped by advances in telemedicine and virtual consultations. These platforms have become increasingly important, especially in the wake of global challenges that restrict physical access to healthcare facilities.

Through telemedicine, individuals can connect with healthcare professionals from the comfort of their homes, receiving expert advice and guidance on managing neck pain. This accessibility ensures that even those in remote areas can benefit from professional consultations, making healthcare more inclusive and widespread. Virtual consultations also facilitate follow-up care, allowing patients to discuss progress and adjust treatment plans without the need for frequent in-person visits. This continuity of care is crucial for effective neck pain management, as it fosters consistent support and adaptation to emerging needs.

Technology's role in self-care extends to the development of apps designed for tracking progress and symptoms. These apps allow individuals to log their daily activities, pain levels, and exercise routines, creating a comprehensive digital record of their health journey. By visualizing this data, users can identify patterns and triggers, gaining insights into what exacerbates or alleviates their neck pain. This self-awareness is invaluable, as it enables individuals to tailor their routines and interventions based on personal experiences. Furthermore, many of these apps offer reminders and motivational prompts, encouraging users to stay committed to their neck care routines. This blend of technology and personal accountability represents a shift towards more personalized, data-driven healthcare solutions.

Personalized medicine is poised to revolutionize neck pain management by tailoring treatments to individual needs. Advances in genetic research have paved the way for exercise programs that consider genetic predispositions, allowing for more precise interventions. By understanding the genetic factors that influence muscle composition and connective tissue resilience, healthcare providers can design exercise regimens that maximize benefits while minimizing risks. This tailored approach enhances the effectiveness of treatments and reduces the likelihood of injury.

Personalized medicine acknowledges that no two individuals are the same, offering bespoke solutions that respect and optimize each person's unique physiology.

Looking ahead, the integration of artificial intelligence (AI) in developing personalized treatment plans holds immense promise for neck pain relief. AI algorithms can analyze vast amounts of data, identifying patterns and correlations that may elude human observation. This capability can lead to the creation of highly individualized treatment protocols, predicting which interventions are likely to yield the best outcomes for each patient. AI can also assist in monitoring adherence to prescribed routines, providing feedback and recommendations in real-time. As AI technology continues to evolve, its application in neck pain management could lead to unprecedented levels of customization and precision, transforming the way we approach treatment and prevention.

These emerging trends and technologies signal a future where neck pain management is both proactive and personalized. By embracing these innovations, individuals are empowered to take control of their neck health, guided by data-driven insights and expert support. The journey towards a pain-free life is no longer a solitary endeavor but a collaborative effort between individuals and technology, paving the way for a future where neck pain is not just managed but effectively mitigated. As we stand on the brink of these advancements, the potential for improved outcomes and enhanced quality of life is both exciting and profound.

8.5 YOUR JOURNEY CONTINUES: ENCOURAGEMENT FOR ONGOING HEALTH AND WELLNESS

As you move forward on the path to neck pain relief, consider this a lifelong commitment to your well-being. The journey doesn't end with the alleviation of pain; it extends into the continuous nurturing of your health. Developing and maintaining healthy habits is paramount, not only for recovery but for sustaining a life of vitality and resilience. Picture your health as a garden that requires regular care—watering, weeding, and tending to ensure it flourishes over time. These habits, once formed, become second nature, seamlessly blending into your daily routine.

Setting new health goals is an effective way to prevent complacency and keep your motivation alive. Goals act as benchmarks, guiding you towards greater achievements and reminding you of the progress you've made. Consider what aspects of your health you'd like to improve or maintain, and set specific, measurable objectives. Perhaps it's increasing your flexibility, enhancing your strength, or integrating more mindfulness practices into your day. Whatever they may be, these goals provide direction and purpose, encouraging you to continue striving for better health.

The interconnectedness of physical, mental, and emotional well-being is undeniable. Each facet supports the others, creating a balanced foundation for a fulfilling life. Continuing mindfulness practices is essential in this regard, promoting mental clarity and emotional stability. These practices help you manage stress, a common trigger for neck pain, and foster a sense of calm and focus. By nurturing your mental and emotional health, you bolster your physical resilience, creating a holistic approach to wellness that extends beyond the physical realm.

Engaging with others who share similar experiences can be incredibly empowering. Sharing your journey, including both triumphs and challenges, fosters a sense of community and connection. Consider contributing your success stories to support groups or online forums. Your insights and experiences can provide encouragement and guidance to others who are on a similar path. By participating in these communities, you receive support and offer it, creating a reciprocal relationship that enriches everyone's experience.

Interactive Element: Reflection Section

Take a moment to reflect on your progress thus far. What healthy habits have you developed, and how have they impacted your well-being? Write down your thoughts and consider setting new goals that align with your vision for continued health. Revisit this reflection periodically, adjusting your goals as needed to ensure they remain relevant and motivating.

Through this ongoing commitment to health, you embrace a proactive approach to wellness. The strategies you've learned become tools in your arsenal, ready to be deployed whenever needed. By integrating these practices into your life, you build a framework for sustained health and happiness. This journey is not just about overcoming neck pain; it's about cultivating a lifestyle that supports your overall well-being. As you continue to explore new avenues for growth and improvement, remember that each step you take is a step toward a healthier, more vibrant you.

A FUTURE FREE FROM NECK PAIN

I have no doubt that you'll inspire everyone around you to take care of their health when they see what you're doing, regardless of whether they have neck pain or not. But if you'd be willing to spare just a few minutes, you'll also help me reach more people who need this guidance in order to manage their neck pain.

Simply by sharing your honest opinion of this book and a little about how it's helped you, you'll help new readers find it and show them that there's more they can do to help themselves than they may have realized.

WANT TO HELP OTHERS?

Thank you so much for your support. I wish you a healthy, pain-free future.

Scan the QR code below to leave your review on Amazon.

CONCLUSION

As we come to the end of our journey together, I want to take a moment to reflect on the core message of this book: neck pain relief is achievable through a holistic approach that combines targeted exercises, lifestyle changes, and mental wellness techniques. By addressing the physical, emotional, and environmental factors that contribute to neck pain, you can create a personalized path to recovery and long-term well-being.

Throughout these pages, we've explored a wide range of strategies to help you alleviate neck discomfort and reclaim your quality of life. From ergonomic workstation adjustments to mindfulness practices and strengthening exercises, each chapter has provided practical tools and insights to support your journey. We've delved into the importance of proper posture, sleep hygiene, and stress management, highlighting the interconnectedness of these elements in maintaining neck health.

It's crucial to remember that there is no one-size-fits-all solution to neck pain. The key is to adapt the strategies outlined in this book to your unique needs and lifestyle. What works for one person may not work for another, and that's okay. By experimenting with different techniques and listening to your body, you can develop a customized approach that resonates with you.

Achieving lasting relief from neck pain requires a long-term commitment to your health and well-being. The practices and habits you cultivate through this book are not meant to be temporary fixes, but rather lifelong tools for maintaining a healthy, pain-free neck. Consistency is key. By integrating these strategies into your daily routine and making them a priority, you lay the foundation for sustained relief and improved overall wellness.

I encourage you to take action today. Start by implementing one or two of the exercises or lifestyle changes discussed in this book. Perhaps it's setting up an ergonomic workstation, practicing deep breathing exercises, or incorporating gentle neck stretches into your morning routine. Small steps can lead to significant improvements over time. Remember, progress is not always linear, and setbacks are a normal part of the journey. Be kind to yourself and celebrate your successes, no matter how small they may seem.

You don't have to navigate this path alone. Engaging with a supportive community can provide motivation, encouragement, and valuable insights from others who are on a similar journey. Consider joining online forums, social media groups, or local support networks dedicated to neck pain relief and overall wellness. Sharing your experiences, challenges, and triumphs with others can foster a sense of connection and empowerment, reminding you that you are not alone in this pursuit.

As you move forward, I want to leave you with a message of hope and empowerment. Having lived with neck pain myself, I know firsthand the transformative potential of the strategies outlined in this book. By dedicating yourself to your well-being and embracing a holistic approach, you can experience significant improvements in your neck health and overall quality of life. You have the power within you to create positive change and reclaim the vitality you deserve.

Before we part ways, I want to express my heartfelt gratitude for choosing this book as your guide on your neck health journey. Your commitment to your well-being is commendable, and I am honored to have played a role in supporting you along the way. Remember, your journey doesn't end here. Continue to explore and expand your knowledge of neck health and wellness. Seek out additional resources, such as websites, apps, or recommended reading, to further enrich your understanding and support your ongoing progress.

You have the tools, knowledge, and resilience to create a life free from neck pain. Embrace the journey ahead with curiosity, compassion, and a steadfast belief in your ability to heal. Your dedication to your well-being will benefit you and inspire others around you. Together, we can foster a community of individuals who prioritize their health and support one another in the pursuit of a pain-free, vibrant life.

Thank you for embarking on this transformative journey with me. I wish you all the best as you continue to nurture your neck health and overall well-being. Remember, every step you take towards self-care is a step towards a brighter, more comfortable future. Keep shining, keep thriving, and know that you have the power within you to achieve lasting relief and vitality.

With gratitude and support, Dr. K.D. Christensen

REFERENCES

Hopler, Whitney. "Famous Quotes on Fitness and Well-Being." Center for the Advancement of Well-Being. Accessed March 26, 2025. https://wellbeing.gmu.edu/famous-quotes-on-fitness-and-well-being/.

Cervical Spine Anatomy https://www.spine-health.com/conditions/spine-anatomy/cervical-spine-anatomy

Tech neck: Effect of technology https://www.mayoclinichealthsystem.org/hometown-health/speaking-of-health/effect-of-technology-on-your-neck

The Effects of Stress on Back and Neck Pain https://www.sandiegospinesurgeon.com/blog/the-effects-of-stress-on-back-and-neck-pain-35634.html

When to seek immediate medical attention for neck pain https://www.health.harvard.edu/pain/when-to-seek-immediate-medical-attention-for-neck-pain

Unearthing the Best Ergonomic Office Chair for Neck Pain ... https://corechair.com/unearthing-the-best-ergonomic-office-chair-for-neck-pain-an-in-depth-look-at-corechair/?srsltid=AfmBOoq6Jr9vgMledxv37jF23k4xKiA6_IMCU_oF0-N69EeZTtWDyz7H

The hazards of excessive screen time: Impacts on physical ... https://pmc.ncbi.nlm.nih.gov/articles/PMC10852174/

Anti-Inflammatory Foods for Optimal Spinal Health https://spinehealth.org/article/anti-inflammatory-foods-for-optimal-spinal-health/

Neck Stretches and Exercises for Pain Relief https://www.webmd.com/fitness-exercise/fitness-neck-stretches

Exercises for neck muscle and joint problems https://www.nhsinform.scot/illnesses-and-conditions/muscle-bone-and-joints/neck-and-back-problems-and-conditions/exercises-for-neck-problems/

Cervical Exercise: https://www.spine.org/Portals/0/assets/downloads/KnowYourBack/CervicalExercise.pdf

EXERCISE: Using a Foam Roller to Relieve Neck Pain https://www.amplifychiropractichv.com/blog/posts/exercise-using-a-foam-roller-to-relieve-neck-pain

3 Ways to Improve Forward Head Posture https://www.spine-health.com/blog/ways-improve-forward-head-posture

Yoga Poses for Your Neck to Stretch and Stimulate https://www.yogajournal.com/poses/anatomy/neck/

Office ergonomics: Your how-to guide https://www.mayoclinic.org/healthy-lifestyle/adult-health/in-depth/office-ergonomics/art-20046169

Pilates for neck pain: 10 exercises to alleviate the discomfort https://www.healthshots.com/fitness/staying-fit/benefits-of-pilates-for-neck-pain-and-best-exercises-to-try/

Neck Stretches and Exercises for Pain Relief https://www.webmd.com/fitness-exercise/fitness-neck-stretches

5 Pressure Points for Neck: Treat Neck Pain Holistically https://www.healthline.com/health/pressure-points-for-neck

Should I Use Ice or Heat for Neck Pain? https://www.healthline.com/health/neck-pain/ice-or-heat-for-neck-pain

Trigger Point Therapy for Neck and Upper Back Pain https://www.painwhisperer.com/trigger-point-neck-upper-back-pain

The Association Between Neck Pain and Psychological ... https://pmc.ncbi.nlm.nih.gov/articles/PMC10066660

Mindfulness meditation to control pain https://www.health.harvard.edu/pain/mindfulness-meditation-to-control-pain

Cognitive Behavioral Therapy for Chronic Pain https://www.va.gov/painmanagement/docs/cbt-cp_therapist_manual.pdf

Benefits of Guided Imagery for Pain Management | Beaumont https://www.beaumont.org/services/pain-management-services/benefits-of-guided-imagery-for-pain-management

The best fitness apps to keep track of your progress in 2023 https://www.womanandhome.com/health-wellbeing/best-fitness-apps/

SMART Goals in Physical and Occupational Therapy https://www.securityhealth.org/-/media/Provider/S-M-A-R-T--Goals-Overview-Writing-Tips-and-Resources_PT-OT-FINAL.pdf

6 Tips to Overcome a Weightlifting Plateau https://www.verywellfit.com/six-tips-to-break-through-strength-training-plateaus-3120744

Why Accountability Is an Important Part of Achieving Your ... https://www.precisionnutrition.com/why-accountability-in-fitness-is-important

Patient success story of upper back and neck pain https://www.pinnaclechirowestfargo.com/patient-success-story-of-upper-back-and-neck-pain-at-pinnacle-chiropractic-and-rehab/

Neck Pain Management: Comprehensive Guide https://persaudlab.jhmi.edu/neck-pain-management-comprehensive-guide

Treatment of Neck Pain: Noninvasive Interventions https://pmc.ncbi.nlm.nih.gov/articles/PMC2271098/

Advances in Pain Medicine: a Review of New Technologies https://pmc.ncbi.nlm.nih.gov/articles/PMC9334973/

Made in the USA
Monee, IL
04 November 2026

67378115R00085